FIT IN BITS

(Staying in Shape When you absolutely, positively, don't have time to stay in shape)

Dr. John Charles Thomas, Ph.D.

Copyright © 2016 by John Charles Thomas.

WHY I WROTE THIS BOOK

My degrees are in psychology and I have spent most of my career in the computer and communications industry. My friends and colleagues there work very hard. Partly, this is because they love their work; the work is challenging and ever-changing. Partly, they work hard because it is a very competitive field. Many companies in the IT industry now have "flex time" which basically means you can work any 70 hours a week you want. These folks are "exempt" which means they are not paid overtime. Many of my other friends and colleagues are academics. They also typically put in 70 hours a week or more. I have seen many of these friends get progressively more out of shape over time, adding inches and pounds as they age. This makes them more susceptible to cardio-vascular disease. More recent evidence suggests that exercise not only makes you thrive physically but also mentally and emotionally. Yet, when the time pressures of commuting and family are added to the overwhelming time pressures of the job, it is much easier to plop down at the end of a very long day with a glass of wine or a couple beers and engage in something sedentary such as watching TV, catching up with Facebook or doing a crossword. They know that staying in shape would be a good thing, but they don't have time, or so they sincerely believe. Or, they may simply not think of exercise as a possibility during "normal" life.

As I see people around me, it is not only people in IT and academics who are incredibly busy. The *majority* of people seem to be skimping on exercise, relaxation, and "down time" due to the combined time pressures of the job(s), family, commuting, and just dealing with the complexity of modern life. Many companies have decided that a good way to reduce their own expenses is to put more burden on the consumer. On the one hand, we have the convenience of on-line shopping but on the other hand, we have to get an account, create a password, learn that the password we chose does not follow the rules for that particular site, lose the password, write email to get a new temporary password, and so on. We spend endless time servicing all our "labor-saving" devices. We don't have to do the dishes "by hand" but we still have to rinse them, reorganize them, put them away, buy the dishwasher, buy the soap, determine who is qualified to fix the dishwasher when it fails (which it invariably will), call and make an appointment, call back when the dishwasher repair person does not show, make another appointment and so on. It is no wonder people often feel too pressed for time for sufficient exercise. On top of that, at day's end, people *feel* exhausted from the press of modern life and often assume that it is a signal that they need rest. Indeed, it typically would have been precisely such a signal through most of our evolutionary history.

I have always played and enjoyed sports. Not only do sports provide one way to help stay in shape, but they have also provided a lot of metaphorical material for my professional work. These sports provide you a lot more fun if you are in shape. Over the course of my long career, I invented ways to stay in shape when pressed for time. I share these in hopes that you can be healthier, happier, and think better. You may also be led to enjoy sports which, in turn, will provide you additional motivation to stay healthier in a virtuous cycle.

Why You Should Read This Book

This book will help you stay youthful and healthy. If you follow the suggestions in this book intelligently, you should be able to increase your cardiovascular health, keep your bones and muscles stronger longer, improve your mood and improve your thinking. Because you yourself are in a better mood, you may find your social relationships improving as well. You may actually do *better* at your job by getting more fit. You will also provide a good role model for your children and grand-children as well as your co-workers and colleagues.

I have tried to strike a balance between providing a complete accurate description of all the suggestions and exercises in this book and keeping you awake long enough to read the entire book. Indeed, words are not very well suited for illustrating exactly how a movement is to be made. Instead, you will find it useful to search on youtube for a four videos illustrating the various exercises mentioned in this book. If you look for "Fit in Bits" and my name, you should find them relatively quickly.

DEDICATION

This book is dedicated to two brave souls: Cathy Wolf and Avery Grace Kalk. Cathy has been a colleague in Human Computer Interaction for many years. More than two decades ago, she was diagnosed with ALS. Now completely paralyzed except for her eyes, she nonetheless writes poetry, is active politically, and does research on brain-computer interaction.

Avery was born with very different heart. As of her third birthday, she already had nine major operations. After her last major operation, her heart stopped for twenty minutes before they were able to hook her up to a heart lung machine. The doctors repeatedly gave up on Avery but her family never did. Nor did Avery herself. She now fights every day to regain her speech and control of her limbs.

Your mobility is a great and wonderful gift. Do not squander it. Use it.

ACKNOWLEDGEMENTS

I would like to thank my many dedicated, hard-working colleagues in Human-Computer Interaction and more generally to hard-working people throughout our society. Many have provided inspiration for the need for this book as well as ideas for approaches to help stay more fit. I would especially like to thank my wife, Wendy Kellogg, and my good friends and colleagues Terry Roberts and Bonnie John for many suggestions and corrections.

TABLE OF CONTENTS

Chapter 1. The Importance of Staying In Shape.

A Word of Caution

Before embarking on any exercise program, you should check with the person or persons responsible for your health. Although most of the exercises recommended in this book are far less vigorous than running or swimming, say, you still want to make as sure as possible that your body is ready, particularly if you have been doing mostly sedentary things for years. You will feel more confident in doing any exercise program if you have been checked out by your doctor.

The second word of caution is to use common sense. I cannot cover the entire world of what constitutes common sense, but I will give a few examples. I may say that juggling provides a good exercise for your coordination. And so it does. I may fail to mention that you are better off juggling balls designed for juggling than juggling running chain saws or poisonous snakes. Use your common sense! Similarly, an excellent exercise for your quads is to sit with your back against a wall and your thighs parallel to the ground while your shins are at right angles to the floor. This will help keep your legs strong. But you obviously want to make sure that the wall will support your weight. Do not use this exercise against a tree with poison ivy vines on it. Do not try this exercise against an electrified fence. Do not try this against the "flats" that are used in drama productions. I cannot be there with you in every circumstance so I assume that you will use your common sense in choosing the time, circumstances, and props for these exercises. I apologize to the vast majority of you who do not really need such warnings.

The proper circumstances for exercise apply to the social as well as the physical situation, though probably far less than you might think. If you are walking in the neighborhood, you may imagine that the neighbors will think you are nuts if you exercise your upper body while you walk. Chances are that they will not think any such thing. First of all, they have their own concerns and hard as it is to imagine, they are much more concerned with their own lives than with yours. Second, if they notice you at all, they will much more likely think you are exercising than that you are nuts. However, if you go to a job interview and during the interview, you squat against the wall to build up your quads, you are on your own. *Some* interviewers might be quite impressed with this move, particularly if you have been practicing and can hold the position for a count of 100. But I cannot predict which ones those will be. The bottom line is that you have to use your common sense in applying the exercises in this book (just as you do in applying knowledge in every other aspect of life).

Finally, the last "caution" is that, while this book contains an awesome array of good ways to stay in shape, you need not *limit* your exercise program to the examples given here. You need to cultivate the habit of looking at the world creatively with an eye to what will work in your circumstances to help you reach your fitness goals. You may well invent many good exercises that are useful for *you* that I never thought of.

CARDIO-VASCULAR HEALTH

The positive effect of exercise on cardio-vascular health is probably pretty well known by everyone at this point, but you might want to check out WebMD at http://www.webmd.com/ heart-disease/guide/exercise-healthy-heart or take a look at http://www.heart.org/HEARTORG/HealthyLiving/ PhysicalActivity/FitnessBasics/American-Heart-Association-Recommendations-for-Physical-Activity-in-Adults_UCM_307976_Article.jsp#.Vql_ssf0RcY

Basically, cardio-vascular exercise benefits the heart but also the arteries and even adds mitochondria in the cells. Naturally, as in everything else in life, it is possible to overdo training, but if you are already running too many marathons, this book is not really aimed at you (though you are welcome to read it for the insightful insights and the catchy catch phrases). If, on the other hand, you are pretty much a sedentary worker with little cardio exercise in your life, then you want to ramp up slowly and check with your physician.

MUSCULAR HEALTH

Basically, there are age-related losses in muscle strength that typically occur as adults age. *However,* many investigators believe that this observed decrease has much more to do with an increasingly sedentary lifestyle typically associated with aging than with any irreversible and intrinsic process. In the age of Google™, you can verify this for yourself, but here is a nice summary by Len Kravitz, Ph.D. at the University of New Mexico, "The Age Antidote" (http://www.unm.edu/ ~lkravitz;Article%20folder/age.html. You can also check out the 2002 review by Williams, G., Higgins, M. and Lewek, M. "Aging skeletal muscle: physiologic changes and the effects of training," in *Physical Therapy,* **82**(1), 62-68. Basically, it appears that the initial increases in apparent strength that come with weight training are primarily neural and these are followed with continued increases in actual muscle strength. These increases in strength can occur at any age. As people age, however, there may be, for some folks, reasons that weight lifting regimens designed for younger people may be less appropriate. Check with your medical provider, obviously, before embarking on a program and have them work with your personal trainer.

By the way, there is a bonus to having better musculature. You look better! There is another bonus. You are stronger! Did I mention that greater muscle mass also means you burn more calories even while you are just giving a lecture, say, or watching *Star Trek* re-runs?

BONE HEALTH

Not only do weight bearing exercises such as running, hiking, weight lifting, tennis, and aerobic dancing increase or maintain muscle strength; they also help keep your bones stronger throughout life. Becoming brittle in old age and falling down and breaking bones is painful, inconvenient, and potentially life threatening. If only there were something that could be done to help *prevent* or *slow down* osteoporosis. Oh, wait! There is! Weight bearing exercise! See, for instance http://nof.org/exercise or http://www.niams.nih.gov/health_info/bone/Bone_Health/Exercise/default.asp

BRAIN HEALTH

It seems to me that if exercise means that you are more likely to live longer, stay stronger, and be less likely to break bones, that would be *plenty* of reason to exercise! But more recent studies seem to indicate that not only is exercise good for your body; it is good for your brain as well! Imagine! Here's a nice summary article by Heidi Godman: http://www.health.harvard.edu/blog/regular-exercise-changes-brain-improve-memory-thinking-skills-201404097110. If you would like to dive a little more deeply into the underlying mechanisms, you might take a look at the article, "Exercise builds brain health: key roles of growth factors cascades and inflammation" by C.W. Cotman, N.C. Berchtold, and L. Christie in *Trends in Neuroscience,* October, 2007, Volume 30, number 9, pages 464-472.

MOOD HEALTH

There are now many studies showing that exercise tends to promote a better mood, both in the short term and also there is a longer term effect. You can easily verify this from your own experience, but if you want to check it out first, feel free to google on your own. One starting point might be the article, "The Exercise Effect" by Kirsten Weir in the *American Psychological Association Monitor,* December 2001, Volume 42, number 11, page 48. If you prefer, you could check out what WebMD has to say http://www.webmd.com/depression/guide/exercise-depression.

To summarize, exercise is awesome! And, if you can ramp up to regular and vigorous exercise nearly every day, great! That is certainly what I have tried to do for years. If there are times when you cannot make the time to save your life though, this book has tips to keep you from just totally disintegrating. See? Your mood is already improving!

CHAPTER 2. PEOPLE R PREST 4 TIME.

We live in the age of "labor-saving devices," speed, and efficiency. Or, so we are told. In point of fact, many people have to work long hours without overtime pay, work more than one job, or commute long hours. Labor saving devices do save time — when they work. But when they stop working, it requires a lot of time to find out how to fix them and then actually fix them. And, of course, you have to work more hours to get the money to buy the devices and then to repair them. In addition to all the time that people spend actually working, there are also countless distractions such as Facebook™, Twitter™, e-mail, television, and so on.

Parenting is tremendously rewarding. However, it is also tremendously time-consuming. This too has changed considerably since my own childhood. Typically, when I got home from school, I would head out to play with my friends. We played basketball, football, hide and seek, baseball, went biking or played board games. Almost all of it was without adult supervision. Today, many parents spend hours driving their kids to dance school, little league team, etc. I also see many parents wait with their kids for the school bus. If my parents would have waited with me at the school bus stop, I would have been *mortified.* And, the same goes for any one of my childhood friends.

So here we have a situation. Few people today have jobs that require much physical exertion at all. Those job that do require physical exertion put imbalanced stress on the body. They often wear out certain joints. Others build tremendous muscle strength in certain groups while ignoring others. Certainly, a sales clerk who is on their feet all day will feel justifiably tired at the end of the day, and they have been on the go, but they are unlikely to have done enough heavy lifting to prevent osteoporosis or keep their heart in shape.

Those who have sedentary jobs like many of my academic friends have it even worse. They sit for endless hours in front of a computer typing, scrolling, and clicking. A successful academic career requires dedication, but meanwhile, their bodies slowly but surely suffer. Sadly, most of the *other* activities that people engage in are *also* sedentary. Commuting, attending PTA meetings, helping kids with homework — these further age you prematurely.

Here's the thing. If you continue along the path of spending no time in systematic exercise, you will not reap the benefits of exercise. People have known for millennia that exercise leads to a healthier, happier life, but now science has confirmed it. We even understand many of the mechanisms. We are learning more about these all the time, but this book does not focus on that ever-growing body of knowledge. This book assumes that you *know* exercise is good for you but that you feel you do not have time to exercise.

In the best case scenario, you would re-think your priorities, see a physician, and engage in a comprehensive life long program of exercise. This book can help you supplement that exercise program by making use of the many little lost moments that occur in daily life. Or, if you cannot persuade yourself to engage in a regular exercise program, you can still gain some considerable fitness by following the philosophy and techniques of this book.

In the following chapters, I offer many examples of how daily life, even in its gray and sedentary moments, provides opportunities for some kind of useful exercise. Expand on these ideas with your own creativity. The point is to stretch, use your heart, use your muscles, and practice your balance and coordination.

CHAPTER 3. THE ADVANTAGES OF THE EXERCISES IN THIS BOOK.

If you have the opportunity to pursue a regular program of exercise, so much the better. For example, maybe you lift weights three times a week for an hour and play tennis singles four or five times a week. Wonderful! However, the exercises in this book, whether undertaken as a supplement to such a routine or as the major part of your exercise program, offer many advantages in terms of convenience, money, and time.

CONVENIENCE.

For the most part, the exercises outlined in this book can be undertaken regardless of the weather. You do not need to wait for winter or summer. You do not need to worry about rain. You do not have to find a golf course or tennis court. You do not have to be at home to engage in most of these exercise. You do not have to get into special clothes or get out special equipment. You can use your own body, your physical surroundings, and in some cases, your friends and family to provide all you need for your exercises.

There is another and more subtle aspect of convenience here. If you are sick, injured, or just not feeling your best, you may call off a tennis match or not participate in a soccer game. You may feel discouraged about going to the gym and not being able to do your regular weights and repetitions. But the exercises in this book can be gradually modified in terms of effort and duration to suit whatever your current state of health.

MONEY

Most organized sports cost money. Some, like polo and sailing require considerable money. Others, like golf and tennis require a moderate amount of money. Still others, like running, require very little capital outlay. The exercises in this book are basically free.

TIME

Not only do these exercises not take up a huge block of time; the time they do take can be whenever it is convenient for you and can be done in any length of time. If you set up a tennis game, you are going to want to play for at least an hour. If you play a round of golf, it will take at least three to four hours. You can do the exercises here for three seconds, three minutes or three hours depending on what else is going on in your life. You need not even know ahead of time. If you are waiting for someone, for example, you can exercise until they get there. If that turns out to be only one minute, they you will have exercised for one minute. If it turns out that you had to wait twenty minutes, then you will have exercised for twenty minutes.

CHAPTER 4. YOU DO NOT HAVE TO WALK ALONE.

When I managed the speech synthesis group at IBM Research, I sometimes *ran* my group meetings. And, by "ran my group meetings", I mean that we physically ran during the meetings. Of course, this only works if your group happens to all be capable and interested in running. I happened to be lucky. But even when the various people I interacted with were not runners, it was very often the case that people were quite willing to *walk* during meetings. Meetings where the participants walk generally have a different (and better) flavor to them than meetings where everyone is sitting down. In my experience, people tend to be more creative and less political when walking. I'd love to see further empirical work along these lines. I am certainly not the only executive or manager who feels that walking meetings are better however. The Huffington Post provides an article with further pointers in the April 9, 2015 issue.

It turns out that many people actually *like* to walk. It is generally just tradition that keeps people sitting down for meetings. Granted, some types of meetings require working with artifacts, or using technology in ways that are currently hard to replicate in an outdoor setting. Not every meeting is of that ilk however, and many meetings in academia or industry can be at least partly walked.

Not only do many people in business and academia enjoy walking; surprisingly, so do many of your friends and relatives! The next time you have a Thanksgiving feast with your extended family do not *assume* that absolutely everyone wants to sit down and watch football games for three or four hours. Everyone may assume that no-one else wants to walk so no-one bothers to ask.

If you *ask*, you will almost always find takers. Bring your walking shoes! You can become one of those families that walks after a Thanksgiving feast.

If you drive your kids to the store, they are quite likely to plug in to their own electronic entertainment. If you walk together, yes, they might still do that. But they are much likely to get involved in a conversation with you if you walk together. This is especially true when they are small. If you get into the habit of walking together when they are young, they are likely to continue the habit beyond young childhood. Consider walking to the store. You might have gotten into the habit of driving when you lived far away from stores but now perhaps you are living where walking to the store might be feasible.

Walking is a wonderful exercise for the body since it elevates heart rate, uses numerous muscles, requires balance, and is weight bearing. I am convinced that it also exercises the brain in several ways. For example, as you walk forward, you see things in the distance. Your brain unconsciously generates thousands of hypotheses about the objects and relations in your field of view. As you walk, your brain gathers more information allowing it to confirm or disconfirm those hypotheses. In other words, you are "fine-tuning" your visual information processing all the time while you are walking. Furthermore, your senses of smell, sound, touch, and kinesthesia are all involved in walking. Walking allows you to keep correlating all these senses as well. You perceive that you are about to walk up a slight incline. Now, you reach the incline and your body feels different as it walks up the incline. You *think* you hear the song of a cardinal but you do not see a cardinal. As you walk closer, it takes flight and you see the telltale red feathers and crest of a male cardinal. Walking thus provides an *integrative* opportunity for your brain. That is in sharp contrast to much of what you see on television. On television, you are seeing one cut shot after another without your providing any motion. In commercials, you may be seeing a long sequence of seemingly unrelated shots, each designed to capture your attention. These snapshot experiences must *de-correlate your brain!* Walking provides an antidote.

All walking is good exercise, and walking through nature is even better. There have been several studies indicating that walking in a natural setting provides mental health benefits. If you reflect on your own personal experience, you can probably verify this but if you would like to take a look at some references, you might check out *The Atlantic,* June 30, 2015; or *Ecopsychology* "Examining group walks in nature and multiple aspects of well-being: A large scale study," Ecopsychology, DOI: 10.1089/eco. 2014.0027. A study in Ann Arbor compared walking in the Arboretum with walking on the streets and found cognitive benefits in the former (Marc Bergman, John Jonides, and Stephan Kaplan, *Psychological Science,* "The cognitive benefits of interacting with nature," **19** (2), 1207-1212. Even if you are not persuaded by empirical study, just try it yourself!

By the chapter title, "you need not walk alone," I also mean something else. Not only can walking often be done as a social activity, it can also provide the basis for a complete upper body strength workout. The basic principle is that you can use one group of muscles in your body to provide the counterforce to work another group of muscles. For example, as you walk, you can flex your right arm (using your biceps) while resisting with your left arm (by using your triceps). You can vary the balance of the leverage between the two arms by varying the position of where your left and right hands meet. You may want to repeat this, through the full range of motion, 20-30 times. You can also vary the angle that your right forearm makes with your body. You can hold your right forearm next to your belly, or in line with your hips or slightly outside. By varying this angle, you can work your biceps more thoroughly. Of course, then you switch hands, this time exercising your left biceps and your right triceps. If you want to really build muscle, you can do three sets of these exercises on each side.

I realize that because of differences in the backgrounds of various readers, some of the descriptions of exercises may not be enough to allow everyone to visualize the exercises exactly. For that reason, I have provided free videos that enact most of the exercise suggestions shown here on youtube. If you go to http://www.youtube.com and search for "John Thomas" and "Fit in Bits" you will find a number of videos that will illustrate the various moves in this book much more clearly than I can explain in words. In particular, most of the exercises in this chapter can be found in "Fit in Bits 2" on youtube.

Of course, this same basic principle can be applied to other muscle groups as well. Here are just a few examples. You push your hands against each other in front of your chest to work your pectoral (chest) muscles. You can make small circles, large circles, and vary the plane and positioning of the circles in order to work these muscles in different ways. You can make circles in front of your belt line, in front of your diaphragm, in front of your chest or in front of your face (and everywhere in between). You can alternate clockwise circles with counter-clockwise circles.

Similarly, you can lock the fingers of your two hands together and try to pull your arms apart thus working your back muscles. Again, you can vary the size of circles, the positioning, and the angle of the circles in order to work the muscles of your upper back from various angles. I recommend starting with one set of 10-20 reps working up to three sets of 20-40 reps. At first, doing these exercises will require a little bit of conscious attention on your part, but these moves are not complicated and very soon you can do these exercises quite easily without much attention at all.

Naturally, as with all exercise programs, you need to do two important things. First, you should check with your physician before increasing your exercise regimen. Second, you need to consider the space around you as you do exercises. For example, if you are making large circles with your elbows extended, make sure you do not bump your elbows! You wouldn't think I would have to write that in a book, but sometimes people have been known to overlook the obvious.

Of course, if you spend enough time walking, at some point you will be tempted to run. If your body is ready for it, running can be an excellent exercise as well. I personally enjoy running on nature trails, along lakes and rivers, and along the beach. Running around a track (or any of these venues) allows for a social interaction as well. Run with a friend; run with a small group; run with a large group. This makes it all more fun. But sometimes you may find yourself running around a track alone. And, even though you are doing something great for your body, you may be worried about all the other twenty things on your to-do list. One way I found useful to deal with that is to use the track as a brainstorming partner. I think of a problem that I am trying to solve. Then on lap one, I think of all the words that are relevant to the problem beginning with "A." Say, to take a random example, that I am thinking about how to publicize an ebook. What begins with "A" that is potentially relevant? I might think of the following: Advertising, Ambassadors, Agents, Attention, Airline lounges, Airline Gates, Automobile showrooms, Auto Rental Car waiting lines. Or, I could take a more "far-out" approach. I think of "armored armadillos" How does that relate? Because people are so bombarded with e-mail, TV ads, web pop-ups and so on, that as a defense, they (and I!) develop a kind of hard shell of armor so they basically fail to pay any attention to anything that they do not already know. Hence, if someone is already famous (or recommended by a friend) they may pay attention; otherwise, not so much. By this time, I am starting the next lap and think about ideas beginning with "B" such as Bulletin Boards, Bragging, Baseball Games, Baseball Cards, Brochures, etc.

An alternative is to think of relevant ideas starting with numbers; for instance, you can start with "one" for the first lap, "two" for the second lap and so on. Anyway, thinking of ideas in this way allows you to keep track of your laps and allows you to do "work" at the same time you are exercising.

CHAPTER 5. SOMETHING THERE IS THAT LOVES A WALL.

I love a wall. Why? Because a wall, at least a *good* wall, supports your weight and resists your push. Let's say that you find yourself stuck at the airport because your flight is delayed a half hour. Or, perhaps the plane is not delayed but you were unsure about traffic so you ended up getting there and through security and to your gate with forty five minutes to spare. You see that sturdy steel, brick or concrete wall over there? That can be an exercise partner for you! (Once again, to see these exercises illustrated, please visit www.youtube.com and search for "John Thomas" and "Fit in Bits." The exercises in this chapter are found in "Fit in Bits 1").

Of course, the wall does not have to be in an airport. It could be a tree, a bleacher wall, a gym wall, a mall wall. Anything that is safe and sturdy can offer to be your exercise partner. The main trigger is that you are somewhere waiting with nothing to do. Rather than *just* waiting, you can spend the time productively by increasing your strength or flexibility.

Here are five of my favorite exercises that make use of walls. First, you can stand with your back against the wall and lower you body till your thighs are parallel with the floor. Hold to the count of 20,30,40, 50 or more. This is a great exercise to build quad strength (quads are the muscles on the top of your thighs and are useful for walking, running, biking, and help prevent falls when you trip) and endurance as well as improve the strength of your knee joint. Obviously, if you have very weak legs or bad knees, you may find this exercise too difficult. It can be modified simply by not going down so far. I would not recommend going lower than having your top of your legs parallel to the ground but you can stand closer to the wall and have your thighs at an angle to the wall to make this easier.

A way to build your triceps (the muscles on the back of your upper arm that straighten your arm) and deltoids (the muscles at the top of your upper arm that allow you to lift your arm) is to stand upright with your back against the wall and, with straight arms down at your sides, push your arms back as though trying to move the wall away from you. In order to build strength for a golf swing or a tennis stroke, you can stand upright with your body at a slight angle to the wall and push hard in both the backhand and forehand positions. In other words, imagine how you hit a stroke and then position the wall where the ball would be as you would make contact. Then, instead of hitting a ball (or the wall!) you push hard against the wall. You might be surprised how much this regular exercise can help add distance to your drives or snap to your tennis strokes or batting swings.

Stand about two feet from the wall and face it. Push with your hands and rise up on your toes. This exercise can be used to improve the toning on your chest muscles, triceps, and calf muscles depending on the exact positioning. The farther you stand away from the wall, the harder you will have to push and the more you will be using your arms and chest muscles. You can push statically or, you can do a kind of modified push-up against the wall.

Obviously, in all these exercises, you want to check your surroundings to make sure the exercise is safe. For example, do not attempt this exercise inside a polar bear cage. You might slip on the ice. And, you might get shredded by the polar bear. I would not think this warning is necessary, but I read about someone going inside a polar bear cage. Unfortunately, the chap is dead so we cannot discover the thought process underlying that decision.

You can also use a wall to stretch your Achilles tendon (this is the large tendon on the back of your lower leg that is important for walking, running, and jumping). Stand about a foot away and put the toes of one foot up onto the wall while your heel is on the floor. Slowly stretch your body forward. Stretch one foot to the count of 40-80 and then the other foot. When, I say "count" I mean silently and about one count per second. Counting by ones. Again, I mention this, not because of *you* the current reader. I mention this in case you give it your Uncle's sister's brother-in-law who might be tempted to count by twenties and won't get much out of the exercise or your baby-sitter's aunt's cousin who might count by 1/1000ths and miss dinner.

Of course, while these exercises all provide benefits, the more major benefit is to stop looking at a wall as just a wall. Instead, think of a wall as a resource for you that can be used in many ways. One important way it can be used is as an exercise partner. And so can many other objects in your environment.

Now, some of you may be saying to yourself: "But what about germs? Wouldn't there be *germs* on a wall in the airport?" Yes, germs do live there. And, there are about a thousand times that many germs on the handrails on the escalators and moving sidewalks at airports, not to mention the straps on the transits, the hands of the flight attendants, the seat backs and stereo controls, the door handles in the restrooms, your luggage, the handles of the overhead bins, and the recirculated air on your flight. Whether or not you spend a few minutes helping your body stay healthy with exercise or not, if you are flying, you should wash your hands early and often!

And, some of you might be saying, "Won't I look funny doing exercise in the airport? I'll be the only one!" Excellent! Then, these wall-based exercises can serve *two* purposes. Not only can they enable you to stay young, flexible, and strong. They also serve as "shame-attacking exercises." Typically, you have to go pay hundreds of dollars to a psychotherapist to advise you to do things of this ilk in order to overcome your fear of being different, being unpopular, etc. Now, for the modest price of this book, you can not only get fit physically, you can use the same book to help you get fit *mentally*.

"But what if someone asks me what I'm doing?" Excellent! What a wonderful opportunity that offers! Of course, to be honest, the chances of that actually happening are less than winning the Irish Sweepstakes. I have exercised for the last five decades in all sorts of situations and no-one has *ever* asked me why. But you *could* get lucky. You never know. And, if they do ask you, then you should have some fun.

If you have even the slightest of accents, you should use that to your advantage. For example, if you have a slight British accent, and someone queries why your are sitting against the wall, you answer, "I'm British!" Even, better: "I'm British, don't you see?" The person who asked the question will now spend the rest of the day trying to figure out what that really means. Do the British always do this? Are they practicing in order to curtsy for the queen? Is this a side-effect of eating black pudding? Is it a symptom of mad cow disease?

You could really have some fun here. Sadly, I have to admit though that your fantasies about someone even taking note of your exercise program are pretty minimal in most circumstances. I suppose if you do push-ups across the pews in church during the sermon, you might get some questions, but pushing against a wall in an airport or while waiting in line at the DMV? I doubt it. That does assume that you push against a substantial wall. If you push against a bookcase in the library and knock over a whole string of bookcases like a youtube dominos video, you might get a raised eyebrow. The same goes for knocking over row on row of prophesies at the Ministry of Magic. Generally speaking however, if you use a little common sense, you, like me, will go through an entire lifetime without a question about why you are exercising when everyone else is quietly letting their body rot away. I suppose part of the reason might be that people realize at some level that they should be *joining* you in moving their bodies, not questioning your motives.

Chapter 6. The Road Less Travelled.

Frankly, I'm not sure what I meant when I originally wrote this title in the outline, but many ideas invade my head as I read it now. First, every single act in your life does not require absolute "optimization." For instance, if you are in an airport and have already gone through security and have a five minute walk to your gate but the folks won't let you board for 45 minutes, you are *not* obligated to walk directly to the gate and *sit there* for 40 minutes. There may have been a very good reason that your first grade teacher, Miss Wilkins, drummed this obedient behavior into your head. But now that you have graduated from grade school, it is no longer required. You can take a *circuitous* route to your gate, stopping here and there to smell the roses (if there are any) and to build your quads by standing against the walls (if there are any) and by all means *not* sneaking behind any doors that say "authorized personnel only" or "deadly fumes behind this door" or "here there be dragons."

Of course, there are times when it makes sense to arrive somewhere early. It *does* make sense to arrive at the airport early because there is a lot of uncertainty in how much traffic will hold you up on the way there and how long it will take to check in and how long it will take to get through security. Only teeny variability in walking to the gate seems likely. If you *do* get to the gate 40 minutes early, there is very little benefit. Your plane probably seats 256 people. If you arrive there 2/3 of an hour early, they are not going to say, "Oh, wow! Sally has arrived! Let's take off early." Not happening.

By "road less travelled" I also mean that you do not have to use your brief case *only* as a brief case or your backpack *only* as a backpack or your carry-on luggage *only* as carry-on luggage. All of these have weight and all of them have handles. This means that all three can be used for resistance training; i.e., weight lifting. You can do some weight lifting exercises while you're walking or go somewhere en route and do your exercises. In fact, carrying a briefcase "normally" can *cause* "tennis elbow" even if you do not play tennis. It is not good to "hang" weights at arm's length. Instead, do curls and wrist curls and reverse wrist curls while you walk with your briefcase. You can also lift the briefcase out to the side to shoulder height with a straight arm or out in front of you to shoulder height to work your deltoids. You can use your briefcase (or any of these handled weights) for triceps exercises and upright rowing. This assumes, of course, that there is some space for these moves; that the airport is not jam-packed with people.

At first you might feel "odd" doing something that helps you stay strong and live longer. But, it will help you stay strong and help you live longer. When you think about it, doing *those* things registers way lower on the "odd" scale than carrying around a month's worth of office supplies in a rectangular suitcase so you can work (most likely for free) while you are on the plane. In fact, it is *so* odd that many business travelers have switched to using backpacks. But…you are not backpacking. So, it is just as odd to shoulder a random 35 pound selection of papers, electronic devices, drugstore nostrums, head cushions, headphones, entertainment devices, crossword puzzles, pens, pencils, and nutrition-less snacks. It really shouldn't feel odd then to use your backpack to help you stay healthy.

CHAPTER 7. DAMN THIS TRAFFIC JAM.

Needless to say, the most productive thing you can do if you are caught in a traffic jam is curse it. That almost always causes the traffic to disappear as I am sure you've noticed for yourself. After all, why are all those other people on the road when *you* are trying to get somewhere? Of course, there are many variations on the theme. It may not be so satisfying to blame total strangers. Instead, you could criticize your spouse or your kids. Rather than blame your family or the people on the road you could blame politicians in general or the party you don't vote for. Whatever method you pick, the important thing is to raise your blood pressure and release a lot of artery-clogging free fatty acids without burning them up.

Alas, I typically fail at all of these ploys and find myself relegated instead to other behaviors which I will outline here. I do not recommend them for you but I thought you'd just like to know what I do out of idle curiosity.

The best cure is prevention. I minimize time in traffic jams by scheduling my drives to avoid rush hour. I also use public transportation when feasible. If an unexpected traffic jam occurs and I am driving, I might pull off at a rest stop and do something else for a while. In some cases, I avoid traveling by doing telecommuting or teleconferencing.

By the way, if you find yourself sleepy while you are driving, you definitely need to pull over. Sometimes even a five minute (when pulled over) nap will help you stay alive. Besides caffeine, if you are with someone else, the very best exercise I have found for waking up is to play "hot hands" for five minutes. In case you spent your entire childhood playing video games and reading the outlines of great novels to pass that English exam without actually reading any of the great novels, "hot hands" is a game played as followed. The two players stand face to face a few feet apart. One player puts their hands out with their elbows bent at right angles. So does the other player. One player who is "it" has their hands on top with the palms facing down. The second player, who is "crusher" places their hands directly beneath the hands of "it" but with palms up and touching. Now, the "crusher" attempts to swing one or both hands up quickly and then down again to slap the top of the hands of "it." "Crusher" is allowed to flinch or say distracting things, but once they lose contact with the player above, they are committed. If they manage to slap "it" even slightly, they get another turn as "crusher." But if "crusher" cleanly misses "it's" hands, "it" becomes "crusher" and "crusher" becomes "it." This is good for your reflexes in any case, but serves as a really good way to wake you up. Obviously, the game doesn't substitute for a good night's sleep! It provides a temporary fix only. According to my calculations, you are better off staying somewhere short of your destination and sleeping than falling asleep at the wheel and dying. That's my take anyway. If you can't find a motel, sleeping in front of an all-night store might be safer than being somewhere more deserted.

Despite planning and precautions, I am in traffic on occasion or even on long drives with stop and go traffic. If that happens, I find the best course of action is to switch off driving with my wife. Then I can write, do my chair exercises, listen to a book on tape, or watch an imaginary flying monkey whiz along beside the car, being careful to have it avoid trees, road signs, bridges, and so on. If I am by myself and have to drive, and when I cannot pull over, I employ several exercises with the steering wheel.

Remember that I am not recommending that *you* do this. I am just telling you what I do. But despite that, if you decide to try these exercises that I do, completely at your own risk, you need to make sure you are not so strong that you will break your steering wheel. If you *are* that strong, you don't need to be doing the strength exercises in this book! You may or may not need to work on your cardio fitness. I can't say because I cannot see you and I don't know you and I cannot monitor your heart rate. I don't even know whether you are going to buy the book while I am sitting here writing it. I can only say that *I* am not strong enough to break a steering wheel with the exercises I do. I should also say that I do not want to have a car accident. That would not be conducive to fitness. So, I always *put safety first.* What I find is that exercise on long trips helps me stay alert; however, I am concentrating on the surrounding cars, the road, and so on so that whatever exercise I am doing will be stopped instantly if the situation demands.

All of the exercises involving the steering wheel are two handed. Keep both hands are on the wheel, please. I generally push the steering wheel from various positions for a count of 20-30 and repeat that 20-50 times. Then I push both hands up at an angle toward each other and upwards on the same sort of repetition schedule. Then I push my hands down and together. This combination is a good work out for the pectoral muscles of the chest. Since I am alive while I write this, it should be obvious to you that I do all of these in such a way that it does not alter the steering of the car.

I do a similar set of exercises by pulling the hands apart while holding on to the steering wheel. I place my hands closer to the top and pull down or somewhat closer to the bottom and pull up on the steering wheel. I find the steering wheel is also good for a forearm workout. I try to tilt my hands forward, then try to tilt them backwards. I try to rotate them inwards and then outwards. I try to rotate them around the steering wheel as well in both directions.

Of course, I also find it useful on long trips to stop every hour or so, get out and do at least five minutes of stretching, running, and other exercises that are impossible to do in the car (like "hot hands" also known as "flinch" or "red hands"). It may take me a little longer to get to my destination but I feel so much better. Meanwhile, while actually driving, I also try to keep my legs active. The feet need to stay where they can quickly be applied to the brakes, gas, or clutch of course. Notice that if I am writing a book, I am not dead. So, I make sure, first and foremost that I can perform any operation needed to steer or brake the car. I like to contract my quadriceps muscle and hamstring muscles (the large muscles on the back of the upper leg) at the same time to a count of twenty and repeat this about 20 times. I can do a similar trick with my calf muscles working against the muscle at the front of the shin. Finally, I contract my foot muscles with a similar schedule. I can do all this while my feet are in driving position. I believe having my muscles warmed up allows me to react more quickly. It also helps keep me mentally alert. Your mileage may vary so all I am recommending for you is to do what you normally do but more safely.

CHAPTER 8. SHOP UNTIL YOU DROP.

I don't really care much for shopping with two exceptions. I used to like going to a bookstore. For many years, my wife and I kept Borders in business. Slowly, we began buying more books from Amazon and basically that change appears to have put Borders out of business. Sorry about that, folks. So, that's gone except for those few of you who live near Powell's in Portland or some other cool local bookstore.

Then, to some extent, I "enjoy" going grocery shopping because it requires a delicate balancing act among budget, nutrition, taste, buying enough variety to keep life interesting but not so much that most things spoil before being used. The most basic rule of food shopping is to avoid the middle aisles. Or, to paraphrase Michael Pollan, buy actual food; buy things your grandparents would have recognized as food. Things like nuts, berries, fruits, vegetables, fish, and some meat and dairy — these are food. They are tasty *and* nutritious.

Some of these foods, like the fruits and vegetables, cry out a rainbow of color. Your brain has evolved to know that these colors are signs that the food may have really healthful phyto-chemicals for you. The problem is that marketers leverage that evolution to package crap that consists of various combinations of salt, fat, sugar, corn syrup, soy, wheat, and industrial chemical dyes in *packages* that *look* colorful and fool your brain into thinking there is the slightest actual nutrition or taste in those packages. Whatever laws once existed for "truth in advertising" seem to have long ago been replaced by laws that essentially mean, "anything goes." So, drinks may be labelled "All natural healthful fruit drink" and have almost zero actual fruit in them. The phrase "all natural" means nothing. The drink may be called "healthful" despite numerous studies that show high fructose corn syrup to be bad for you. So, for the most part, the labels mean nothing. The nutritional information, in the fine print, does tell you something, although you must bring your reading glasses to the store in order to be able to read it. A single serving of most of this crap will provide all the sugar you should have for the entire day. Did I mention that it probably also has more saturated fat and salt than you need in your lifetime. Okay, I am exaggerating, but not by much.

Anyway, I digress. *What* you buy when you shop is actually important, especially when food shopping. But the point of *this* chapter is that whatever kind of shopping you do provides another opportunity for exercise. To begin with, you need not circle the parking lot fifteen times until you get a spot as close as possible to the store entrance. Park farther away. Better yet, if feasible, do not drive to the store, but walk there with an empty backpack and return with a backpack filled with groceries. That does take time, so I realize many of you will not be able to do that and still fulfill the requirements of your 80 hour work week. But it actually takes *longer* to find a parking space that saves you a fifty yard walk than it does to walk the fifty yards.

Now, when you grab a cart, take a good look at that cart and realize that it constitutes both a cart *and an exercise machine.* You can use the handle of the cart in various ways pretty much the entire time you hold it in your hot little hands. You can hold on to the cart and push your hands down, push them up, push them apart, or push them together. This allows you to exercise four sets of muscle groups for an upper body workout while you are filling up your cart and driving it back to your car. If you have a kid in the cart, so much the better! That provides extra opportunities to exercise your legs, your patience, and your refusal to be bothered by the stares of strangers who will disapprove of your child rearing practices as being too lenient, too strict, or too non-magical. In any case, because your kid has already been brainwashed into thinking fruit poops will cause magical birds, bubbles, and burping bison to appear out of nowhere, steer clear of the middle aisles of the grocery even more assiduously when accompanying a child. Remember: you are the adult. You are the responsible one. You will be the one having your kid living at your house till they are 35 if you destroy their brain and their health now. You know that magical birds are *not* actually going to appear if they eat poopy fruits. No, you will not be able to explain that to your two year old. You are the adult. You are in charge; you will pay the doctor bills. The advertising agency will not. I've tried that route. The "food" inside a lot of the packages costs nearly nothing. The price you pay for the "food" primarily pays for packaging, advertising, lawyers to prevent you from collecting damages, and buying the politicians who agreed to forgo "truth in advertising." So, you need to resign yourself to the fact that your toddler will try to embarrass you into buying them colorful, masterfully packaged poison.

If you generally steer clear of the middle aisles, at some point, your child has a good chance to grow up to be a pre-teen, at which point, you will find yourself going shopping with them for clothes. In most stores geared toward pre-teens and teens, they will play music while you wait for them. Now, you have a choice. You could spend your time sitting down glancing at your watch or texting on your iPhone. Or, you dance! Dancing rejuvenates the body. Of course, it will embarrass your kids. Depending on your mood, you can dance at the other end of the store and pretend not to know them till it comes time to pay. Or, you can simply remind them of how they used to *scream* in the grocery store to embarrass you. You might offer them the choice that you will either dance or scream, but you need to be prepared to back up that (or any other) threat you make to a child. After an hour or so of dancing, and an hour or so of your offering your opinions (that do not matter one small whit), you will be done with shopping, phase one. Phase two will be when your kid gets the reactions of his or her friends and that will determine whether the clothes will be kept or you move on to phase three. Phase three consists of going back to the store and giving you another opportunity for dancing. I really encourage dancing, but if that is too far outside your comfort zone, you can also use the walls of the store to help support your ever-growing exercise habit.

Regardless of whether you are shopping for clothes, groceries, or books, at some point, you will have bags to carry. Here again, you have a choice. You can let these bags hang uselessly at the ends of your limp arms where they do nothing but overstretch your joint and give you tennis elbow, *or* you take the opportunity of walking through the mall, walking back to your car, and walking from your car to your front door as an opportunity for more exercise. Think of these bags as essentially hand-weights. You can do curls, triceps curls, wrist curls, lateral raises, front raises, and shoulder shrugs. In other words, you can pretty much do a complete upper body workout. (If these terms mean little or nothing to you, remember to check out the youtube videos with keywords "John Thomas" and "Fit in Bits"; at this point, you might want to watch Fit in Bits 3). Need I add that since you are *moving* these bags, you need to make sure you do not smash them into an innocent bystander? I suppose I do. Since you are moving these bags, you need to make sure that you do not smash them into an innocent bystander. In fact, do not even smash them into a questionably innocent bystander. Avoiding such crashes does not require a course in quantum mechanics or even Newtonian physics. If you have lived on planet earth for more than a couple years, you can pretty well predict the arc that a bag of J.Crew pants is going to take through space.

Chapter 9. Sitting for Fun and Profit.

Sitting too long is bad for you. I just wanted to say that up front in case you failed to get the memo, log onto Facebook@, look at your e-mail, or got your tweets and twitters twisted. In other words, if you were hiding in a closet for the last few years, you might not have heard the news. Sitting too long (more than a half hour) is bad for you.

But what are you going to do? You might be on an airplane where you are forced to sit. In the olden days, I pretty much walked, stretched, and otherwise exercised my way through long trips. Now, you are expected to stay in your seat (dammit) and not even wait in line for the bathroom. You have to make a beeline for the bathroom and back. And, if you do happen to get there when the toilet is "in use" you have to hope that it is in "in use" for the ways in which a *toilet* is in use and *not* for one of the many ways that a so-called beauty parlor is in use. Seriously, if people need to do a complete makeover, fine, but do it at your seat. No-one cares if you sit at your seat and put on lipstick, comb your hair, shave, polish your nails, put on perfume or aftershave…well, actually, maybe they do. But they mind even more if you take 45 minutes to handsome-ify or beautify yourself in one of the few on-board toilets.

Here's a little arithmetic example to help you figure out your fair share of toilet time on an airline flight. Let's say there are 200 people in coach. Let's say the flight is five hours. You cannot get out of your seat for the first half hour and the last half hour. So that leaves four hours. Now, on that long of a journey, the flight attendants will come by and block the aisles while they serve you drinks, food, and offer extremely overpriced items from their catalogue. Assuming no-one actually buys anything from the catalogue, that leaves about two hours when the aisles are actually clear and you can hit the head. But wait! There's more. If you have a captain who is deathly afraid of death, or worse, lawsuits, then the slightest 15 second jolt of turbulence will put that seatbelt sign on for at least another hour. So, now you are left with basically *one hour* to get to the bathroom, use it and get back. That is 60 minutes. Divide sixty minutes by 200 people and you see that *your share* is only *20 seconds!* So, no, you don't have time to do a makeover. If your significant other will reject you for not doing a 45 minute makeover on a five hour flight, you are better off without them.

Actually, on any given flight, only about half the people are actually human beings who have bladders, etc. The other half are either automata or so spaced out on drugs that they will not need to get up during the flight. You can tell who these people are ahead of time because they always have aisle seats. So, realistically, you probably have 40 seconds for your turn. However the math works out, you are going to be spending most of the flight sitting in your seat.

Of course, airplanes are not the only times you will be more or less "stuck." You may be "stuck" at a meeting, or in a place of worship, or in your car, or in a movie theater, or on a bus, and so on. How do you deal with it? How do you do what you can to stay strong and healthy?

The first thing to do, as explained above, is not to *assume* that you have to be stuck. Not too long ago, I flew a Chinese airline from New York to Beijing and they didn't care at all if I stood up the entire flight! You might well be able to convince people in a meeting that you should all go out for a walk. Often, even if others are sitting, you can stand at the back and pace.

Taking though the worst-case scenario where you really are in your seat for hours, does that mean you have no exercise options? Absolutely not! If your chair has arms, you can exercise your pecs and your deltoids by alternately trying to push the chair arms together and trying to spread them apart. (Again, check out the youtube videos). If you feel the chair arms start to give way or creak loudly, you may need to back off. After the break, try to pick a different chair. That in itself will leap your contribution to the meeting above those of your co-workers who will return like milting salmon to the same spot, time after time.

Meanwhile, another exercise which does not put the chair at risk is to put your hands in your lap…actually just *above* your lap and push your hands together and then alternatively pulling them apart while holding them. This is pretty much the same exercise as above but without the danger of turning the chair into kindling. From the same position, you can do forearm curls and reverse curls. These are excellent exercises for basketball, tennis, golf, softball, and bar fights.

While sitting in a chair offers many opportunities to do an upper body work-out, it also provides an opportunity for a lower body workout. Some of these exercises are actually suggested in the airline magazines. They *know* that forcing you to sit in a chair so long can kill you, especially when the chairs are designed for baby hobbits. So, to help avoid litigation, they put helpful suggestions, complete with diagrams, about things you can do in your chair to lengthen your life. (These do *not* include, as most seven year olds seem to think, kicking the seat in front of you. Kicking the seat in front of you will not prolong your life and may indeed cause it to end rather prematurely, although I think it would be more fair to institute capital punishment on the *parents* rather than on the seven year old kicker. After all, it's not their fault they were born to parents who incapable of instilling any discipline).

Anyway, what you *can* do, which the airlines to not mention, is to simultaneously contract your hamstring muscles on the back of your upper legs and your quads on the top of your upper legs. You can contract both and play them off against each other for twenty seconds. Relax for ten seconds and repeat. If you do this for the entire five hour flight, you will probably burn at least six calories and need to buy pants with larger pant legs within a week. Alternatively, you can use one leg and then the other to try to push your chair back by using your quads. In a similar fashion, you can work your hands against the outside of your knees, pushing in with your pecs while pushing out with the sides of your legs. After doing this twenty times, you can switch and put your hands inside your thighs. You push in with your thighs while pushing out with your hands, thus working your deltoids. You can also just wiggle your legs back and forth quickly without resistance. This set of exercises is good for lateral movement in basketball, hockey, soccer, or tennis and helps with making a stable foundation in golf. You can similarly, contract the calf muscles on the back of your leg and the muscles on the front of your lower leg at the same time. Finally, you can curl and uncurl your toes within your shoes to help keep your feet fit.

Of course, you do not need to be on an airplane to employ these tactics. You can use variants of these in church, at meetings, on a car trip, on the bus, etc. Oh, yes, I know. In the paranoia that befuddles us all, you fantasize that everyone will notice and you will be hauled off the looney bin for taking the time and care to keep yourself alive. The truth of the matter is that the vast majority of the folks in church, meeting, the bus etc. don't really give a hoot about you. Very few, if any, will notice your actions and if they do, they are extremely unlikely to say anything at all. If they do say something, the most likely thing for them to say is, "Hey, you must have read that cool book about how to stay fit by Dr. Thomas, right?"

You may have another objection. You may believe that if you do these exercises you won't be able to pay attention during the powerpoint presentation, the sermon, or your marathon Facebook session. Nothing could be further from the truth. By keeping your blood flowing and sending oxygenated blood through your body, you will not only be healthier in the long run; you are likely to recall more of the presentations, sermons, and 150 pictures of birthday parties and food items on Facebook than you would if you just sat there.

CHAPTER 10. TRAVELING.

I am not talking about carrying the ball while you run down the basketball court. I am talking about what happens after you travel to another place. After reading the preceding chapters, you have undoubtedly figured out how to incorporate some exercise into your daily routine with a minimum of added time. Hopefully, you have even decided that staying alive is *almost* as high a priority as putting in another half hour on that powerpoint presentation or reading yet another journal paper and you have actually started running, biking, hiking or playing tennis as well which may take some time. In either case, going on a trip poses some special challenges.

I have found that it helps to plan ahead. So, when my wife and I travel, we try to go to a hotel with a gym or ask them about a gym nearby. Often we take our golf clubs with us or our tennis equipment and plan to spend some time with one or both of these activities. If packing these is too onerous, clubs and racquets can generally be rented or borrowed on site. But you need to check ahead of time. I have experimented with the tradeoff between an hour's sleep and an hour's workout and for me, an hour of workout is always better. That is, I feel better if I sleep 7 hours and work out 1 hour than if I sleep 8 hours. I feel better if I sleep six hours and work out one hour than if I sleep 7 hours. I feel better if I sleep five hours and work out one hour than if I sleep six hours. And so on. I *suspect* this would be the same for you but I don't really know.

When you go somewhere traveling, there can be many reasons, but chief among them are traveling on business, travel for vacation/pleasure and travel to see family. Hybrids of these have been spotted occasionally but unlike crop hybrids, such hybrids are typically less hearty and prone to disease. In any case, I will deal here only with the pure breeds. You can experiment with the hybrids. Remember to wear gloves.

If you are traveling on business, you *might* be in a position to have some influence over the venue. You often have power to determine the hotel and what you do in your "free time." Clearly then, to the extent possible, choose a venue (or hotel) that affords itself of a beautiful park, river walk, or nature path. If you have any say over the agenda, build in breaks of at least an hour and a half so that you can walk, go to the gym, go sightseeing on foot, etc.

It is also extremely useful to ask for (or pay a slight fee) for a room with a small refrigerator. In some cases, a minibar can be pressed into service, but beware. Some computerized minibars, as I discovered, charge you the microsecond you lift an item up whether or not you consume it. The hotel management says, in effect, "If you touch it, you buy it!" Or, in other words, "We don't want you looking at the *ingredients* of what you are eating or drinking. If you did that, you might well decide that we have nothing but health-ruining crap in the minibar." However you solve the problem, get yourself a fridge, if possible. Then, arrive in time to *walk* to a store and buy yourself some healthful food. This allows many advantages: healthier food, more economical budget, the affordance of a midnight snack even if room service is closed, and, of course, the walk itself. If the store requires a long walk, you will be more comfortable using a backpack.

Often, even if the agenda-meister squeezes every ounce of humanity out of the schedule, there will be some breaks. Go to the toilet and perhaps, grab your coffee, but find a like-minded individual who wants to *walk* while they chit-chat. There are more pointers in the chapter on meetings.

If you are traveling on vacation, you have more control over the venue and the agenda. You owe it to yourself and your traveling companions to choose times and places that allow exercise. In many cases, the vacation can be *built around exercise.* You can backpack, go to tennis camp, or go on a biking tour. Even many "tours" of ancient cities, castles, cathedrals, or movie studios, will involve a lot of walking. If you are forced to stand in line or sit at any point, you can still use the other exercises in this book to burn more calories and further increase your fitness.

If you are traveling to see family, then tell them ahead of time you would be happy to stop on the way in and do some shopping for everyone. This will allow you to buy some healthy food as well as what is on their list. Some families will raise many objections if you try to eat healthy. They are clearly hoping for an early inheritance. One possible ploy is to tell them that you have become vegetarian. Or tell them you have lethal food allergies. While your family may be happy for you to die young, they usually prefer for you not to do it on their premises. Often if the family gathering consists of more than 2-3 people, you can find someone who is happy to schedule a game of golf or tennis or at least go for a walk. Maybe your family dances or tips cows or likes to bale hay. Whatever it is, look for opportunities to help or participate in something besides watching TV or video games. If you must play video games, suggest Wii@ fitness games or Kinnect@.

Be honest and assertive about your preferences for physical activity. If that doesn't work, then lie, but get it done one way or another. Your life is at stake here! If you are visiting *distant* relatives, you can bring your creativity a bit more into play. You can say, for example, that your psychiatrist said you *had* to exercise vigorously at least an hour and a half a day. Or, you could say it is a condition of your parole. These will be harder to pull off with close family, but you possess the smarts to come up with something. "I got this great book on fitness and then I made this crazy bet with a colleague at work that I would do an hour of exercise every day for the next month. It's not so much that I stand to lose $500 dollars if I don't do it. It's more just a guy (or woman) thing." And, since we are on the topic of books for fitness, need I say that you find your own exercise program much easier to keep up when you travel with friends and colleagues if you provide each of them with a certain *gift* for their birthday, Christmas, Hanukkah, Ramadan, Beltane, or Kwanza? Once they have all read the book, your necessity to plot, scheme, and lie shrinks to nothing.

CHAPTER 11. KIDS PLAY THE DARNEDEST THINGS.

And so should you! As people age, they tend to lose their sense of balance. But is this an inevitable and irreversible effect of aging? Or, is it because as people get older their sense of dignity overcomes their sense of fun? If you are an 80 year old couch potato who has not used their sense of balance much lately, I am not suggesting you take up girder walking to regain your childhood sense of glee. But what you *can* do, as a young parent, is play with your kids on the playground and not just watch them while texting on your cell phone or gossiping with the other parents.

Young kids serve as handy exercise partners in a variety of ways depending on their age and size as well as your own level of fitness. When I was younger, I used to put my toddler kids on my back and do push-ups. Infants are not appropriate because they would roll off and bang their heads. Teen-agers are not appropriate for *most* of you because you are not strong enough and most of them would be mortified anyway. You might or might not find this a useful exercise with toddlers who are grand-kids depending on your level of fitness and your blood pressure.

Another exercise that kids about 8-15 months love in my experience is the game of "airplane." You take your shoes off and balance the child with your feet on their hipbones and holding both their hands in yours. You carefully lift them up with your legs. Obviously, you accomplish this only if you are strong enough and coordinated not to drop the kid on the floor. And, by the way, you do this with your kids and grand-kids. I do not recommend doing this with random kids that you see in the park.

Older kids love to swing. You can push them on the swing and this itself can become a form of exercise for you. By varying the precise *manner* in which you impart energy, you can exercise your triceps, your pecs, or your lats. You can even use it as a wrist exercise useful for tennis, golf, baseball throwing or other sports that require good wrist snaps. When they get on the climbing bars, you join them. When they play hide and seek, you seek and hide as well. Often playgrounds have four inch wide planks for borders. These are most often only an inch off the ground and you can practice your balance while your child or grandchild is practicing theirs. If one of them wants to play on the teeter-totter, you can push down on the other end as an exercise for you and to provide fun for them. Or, get on and use your legs. Just do not let the kid plummet to the ground. Plummeting is for sheep, not for children. Your orthodontia bills multiply quickly enough without your causing them to smack their teeth together when they hit the ground.

Young kids are *great* exercise partners because they have not yet learned to be embarrassed or question the appropriateness. If music fills the sonic sphere, kids fill the visual sphere with flailing limbs. And, you can do the same! At least, you can dance with them till about when they become pre-teens. Then, "oh my God, those are my parents" mortification sets in at the slightest provocation. Spirit still fills you, but they would be happier to think of you as full time homework helper, dishwasher, chauffeur, allowance provider, meal maker, house cleaner, and bread winner. Do not fall for this ploy. You are the adult here; not them. Your body still belongs to you. Keep your body young and fit one way or the other.

Taking your kids grocery shopping offers another opportunity for fun and exercise. Most kids love having you drive that grocery cart a little "crazy." Driving it a *little* crazy gives them a *safe* thrill and forces you to exert more force with your muscles by stopping, starting and turning. Obviously, you do this so as to keep your kids and nearby unsuspecting pedestrians safe. The goal is not to add points to your driver's license. (Do they do that for unsafe grocery cart driving? It wouldn't surprise me.) Anyway, if you get kicked out of your local Von's or Safeway by security, you have taken it too far and you need to back off a little when you go to the A&P or Kroger.

If you are in tight quarters like a Costco's Spectacular Saturday Soap Sale , you may have to forgo your San Francisco Car Chase Fantasy entirely. But you can still burn extra calories while pushing the cart forward by trying to push your hands inward toward each other (without actually sliding them) for a count of twenty and then outwards for an equal count. Repeat. Now, maybe you forgot one of the items on your list. Good. Next time, you will bring a written list. So, this allows mental as well as physical exercise. Speaking of which, why do you fail to care about the destroyed property and maimed bystanders in those car chase scenes?

I have also played being a "climbing tree" for my kids and grandchildren and I have seen many other parents do the same. You stand well braced with your legs slightly apart and putting your hands on your hips and let your kids climb you. In a similar spirit, they can wrap their legs around your legs and sit on your feet and then you can walk (albeit with difficulty) around the house. This gives them a fun ride while building strength in your legs. I also held my arm out parallel to the ground and let my kids use the arm as a "chinning bar." I found this rather difficult once they got to be adults. Here, I refer to the British sense of "rather difficult" which in American English means "completely impossible."

If you are lucky enough to live somewhere with access to a lake, pool, or ocean, additional exercise possibilities abound. You can swim with kids on your back or stomach. Need I say that water safety is important? You have to notice if they slide off and catch them before they drown. You can have them hold on to your arms and "drag them" through the water at high speed by turning your body. This provides an especially good exercise for batting, tennis and golf. Most pools have a graduated depth bottom. So you can "run" across the pool in a deeper part than your child to make the race a little more fair. There are also various ways to "throw" the kid in the water. You need to make sure they land in the water and not on another kid, a rope, or the concrete on the side of the pool. You also need to make sure that this is a kid (about 95%) who *love* this treat and not do it with the 5% of kids who find this frigging terrifying. Just because you loved it does not mean that they necessarily will. And, if they hate it, doing it repeatedly will not change their mind, no, not even if you repeat it a *lot*.

CHAPTER 12. MEETINGS: THE GOOD, THE BAD AND THE UGLY.

Does anyone love being in all day meetings? I doubt it. At least, I doubt many people would enjoy the typical meeting. As I may have mentioned already, the Supreme Court has already determined in the landmark case, *Sorebutt vs. The State of Boredom,* that it is legal to have meetings where people do not sit the entire time. In fact, it is now legal to have meetings where people walk, move around, or even run.

So, if you have *any* power or persuasion in the situation, please try to limit sit down meetings and replace them with standing, walking or even jogging meetings. Meet on the golf course. But if you have to have a sit-down meeting for whatever reason, try to avoid just chowing down on coffee and donuts and instead, try to find some like minded people to walk with you while discuss earth shattering topics.

There is something about working together physically that helps people learn to accommodate each other and cooperate better than they typically do when only words are exchanged. In many cases, physical activities provide form and substance to the work of the meeting. For example, in many meetings, one person at a time will give a presentation. Typically, everyone else is supposed to sit still and listen, possibly asking questions later. In many workshops that I have helped organize and run, however, we use a different technique. There are a variety of flip charts with various topics around the room. What these topics are depends on the context. Examples from some of our workshops have included: References, Unresolved Issues, Suggested Patterns, Problems, Stakeholders, Values, Facts, Questions that need to be Answered, Assumptions, etc. Then, before anyone talks, it is made clear to all the participants that it is quite acceptable for people to write down an idea on a post-it note, get up during a talk, and place it in the appropriate place for later discussion.

In one workshop on human computer interaction for international development, we began the workshop outside by cooperatively making a very large map of the world using materials at hand such as stones and sticks. Then, we "arranged ourselves" on the map according to various questions, such as "where are you living now?", "where were you born?", "what is one place you've always wanted to visit?" and so on.

Your situation will be different, but there is almost always some legitimate way to put space and movement into the work of the meeting. Of course, the other thing you can do is to use any of the techniques from Chapter Nine if you find yourself sitting at a meeting. These techniques can be used any time you *have* to sit, but do not assume that you always have to sit in meetings. If you do sit, doing the exercises from Chapter Nine will help you stay fit and also help avoid the embarrassing situation of falling asleep in a meeting. In the long run, it can help you avoid the even more embarrassing situation of *dying* in a meeting and having no-one realize that you have. Compared with these, the embarrassment of wiggling your toes under the table is minimal.

Chapter 13. Hospital.

It is no accident that people wishing to receive services in hospitals are called "patients." In fact, you will also need to be patient if you are waiting there for someone else. But let's consider both of these situations. First, let's imagine that you yourself are a patient. If you are brought in on a stretcher, unconscious and bleeding with multiple compound fractures from a car accident, I am not suggesting you perform jumping jacks.

On the other hand, consider this case. When I played on the high school JV football team, I ran down the field on the kickoff and the person assigned to me missed their block. On the next punt or kickoff the same thing happened. I suspect that guy's coach was none too happy. In any case, on the third go, I got nailed. I had just put my right spikes into the ground when he blind-sided me with a cross-body block that took out my knee. It took awhile for me to realize this.

My coaches came running onto the field immediately. I waved them off saying I was fine and began to run. I took one step and fell on my face. They started back onto the field and I waved them off, insisting I was fine. I took one step and fell on my face. At this point, they ignored my protestations and carried me off the field. When I went to the hospital, I was laid on my back and put in traction for ten days. I was not used to this and it really hurt my back the first night. I asked the nurses for an aspirin but of course, they could not provide one without a doctor's prescription. Around midnight, after I finally fell asleep despite the noise of being right next to the nursing station and the pain in my back, they received permission to give me a sleeping pill so they literally woke me up to give me a sleeping pill.

The point for this chapter, however, is that once I learned that I would be on my back for ten days, I asked my parents to bring in some hand weights. The hospital also gave me a pair of crutches. I worked out my upper body three times a day, using both the hand weights and the crutches even though I was flat on my back. This helped keep up my spirits and it strengthened my upper body which later turned out to be useful for using the crutches. I mainly used the hand weights, but also held the crutches and pushed on the walls at various angles as well. In addition, the hospital staff seemed quite amazed that I didn't need any artificial help to stay "regular." Indeed, exercise has many benefits.

Now, let's say instead that you are there to see a friend or relative. The chances are excellent that you will find yourself waiting by yourself in the "waiting" room. That's why they call it a waiting room. Typically, hospitals and doctors offices have a variety of magazines lying around. These are the magazines from subscriptions that the receptionist bought from their high school student in order to raise money for their senior class play. Ever notice that the magazine subscriptions for such causes are never "National Geographic" or "The New Yorker" or "The Atlantic Monthly." No, they are magazines like: "Avoiding Botulism" and "Sniping for Fun and Profit" and "Lifestyles of Bolivian Curlers Today." While you are sitting waiting to find out whether your relative or friend is okay or deathly ill, reading about famous Bolivian Curlers is not going to reduce your tension all that much. On the other hand, doing some unobtrusive exercises *will* help reduce tension. It will also keep you awake for the long drive home. Because hospital and doctor's appointments are always arranged in the space-time continuum to maximize your *transportation time* as well as your "waiting room" time.

For starters, you can walk. If you know it's going to be awhile, you can walk to the gift shop and buy a $15 dollar bouquet or stuffed animal. (Of course, it will cost you $50 but that's not the point). The point is that walking there and back is a better exercise than reading a magazine or staring into space.

If the time is unknown, you can still pace around the waiting room or use the seated exercises or, if you feel more comfortable, go outside and pace pack and forth right outside the "waiting room." You do not *have* to wait in the waiting room. It is not a law. And, if you are in the waiting room, you do not have to read their magazines. Of course, you may want to impress the other complete strangers by constantly checking your smart phone. This will totally impress them because you are the only person who constantly checks their smart phone. None of them will have ever seen this behavior before so be prepared for those awestruck looks. But if you really want to impress the total strangers, I say some more vigorous exercise is more likely to do it than scrolling through your IM's.

CHAPTER 14. BECOMING A COUCH POTATO SPROUT.

What can be more antithetical to exercise than sitting on the couch watching television? Isn't this the quintessential non-athletic, artery clogging activity? Why not just write this time off as time subtracted from your time here on earth? Why would I even bother to have a chapter alluding to couch potatoes in a book about staying fit?

I'll tell you why. Because even though it is true that you would be far better off playing golf, tennis, running, or lifting weights than watching television, if you must binge watch for hours at a time or even catch a half hour a week of Gilligan's Island, there are some things you can do to try to minimize the damage you are doing to your body.

First, and most importantly, I have discovered that most television systems work *even when you are walking around the room!* It took me many years to figure this out because they never mention it in the manuals, right? They will tell you how to hook up the cable and the stereo and the Bose system and the Blu-Ray player, but never do they mention that you can actually watch TV from a standing or walking position. Now, I will be the first to admit that there are limits to this general approach. If you walk out of the room containing the TV, you may be able to hear the TV but not see it. And, if you walk out the front door and down the block, you probably will not see or hear the program. However, if you pace back and forth, walk around in a circle or dance while you're watching, you will still be able to keep track of what is going on pretty well. For more variety, and if you have space to do it safely, you might try mimicking the actions of some of the people on television.

The feasibility of doing this depends on the nature of the show as well as the particular episode. For example, if you are watching two people conversing, you might try to copy their gestures. If you are watching Mission Impossible, you may find jumping out of a moving airplane onto a high tension wire and back-flipping beneath a slicing Samurai sword fails to improve your general health. You have to use your judgement here. Similarly, if Grey's Anatomy is your cup of tea, I do *not* recommend that you actually *try* the delicate and potentially fatal (but potentially life-saving) brain surgery on your family members. The idea here is not to win a "Darwin Award," (Based on Darwin's survival of the fittest, these awards are handed out to people who do incredibly stupid things and end up out of the gene pool). but rather to use what is happening on the TV as inspiration for exercise. And, when I say "exercise" in this context, I mean "movement."

You may do a little of this quite naturally already. For example, if you are watching a three-D movie and you see bats flying at you, you duck, whether they are the mammalian variety or the Louisville slugger variety. Your options are not limited to moving around the room and bobbing and weaving however.

Another trick is to use something other than a couch to sit on. For instance, you might try one of those posture balls. This at least will require you to use your core and practice your balance. Another option is to use television time for stretching. In fact you can even stretch during commercials. Commercials allow you plenty of time to stretch muscles *throughout* your body and not, as is popularly believed, time to stretch your legs to the refrigerator for another chunk of cheesecake and another pint of Pinot.

Another possibility is to use small hand weights, or to squeeze a rubber ball while watching. If you play tennis, baseball, or golf, for example, spending time squeezing a rubber ball (or grip trainer) or even the sides of the couch for a half hour a day will do wonders for your game. If you spend your non-TV time typing on the computer, it's even more important to use something for grip strength. Typing and using the mouse does require muscle use, but sadly, not enough to really keep your circulation going so you may fall prey to carpal tunnel syndrome. If you don't have a towel, a couch handle, a rubber ball, or a grip trainer handy, you can always attempt to open a jar of pickles. The design of pickle jars actually prevents them from being opened without high explosives, but the attempt can be useful for improving your grip.

While we are on the subject of sliding joints (which is what your wrists are), do not neglect your ankles. Have you ever had a sprained ankle? Well, it is no fun! So, while you are watching "Reality (nod, nod, wink, wink) TV," circle those ankles! Circle them in synch twenty times clockwise and then twenty times counter-clockwise. Then, you can circle them toward and then away from each other as well. After that, try flexing your foot so that the toes go up toward your knees and then down away from you. Repeat that twenty times as well. You should execute these moves with your feet well off the floor in order to bring your abs into play as well.

Obviously, some of the exercises in other parts of this book are equally applicable here. For instance, you can watch TV while sitting against the wall, with your thighs parallel to the floor and your shins perpendicular to the floor. At first, you can only manage this for a few moments, but eventually, you'll be able to hold this position for longer. Shake it out and repeat. Maybe this is another good time to remind readers that you need to listen to your body. If sitting against the wall this way causes you knee pain, then, don't do it. In the same way, if banging your head against the wall causes you head pain, then do not do that either

(I haven't suggested anywhere that that is a good exercise by the way).

But let's get back to walking. Not only can you walk around the room while you watch television; you can walk and do a complete upper body workout in the space of a half an hour. Chapter four explains these exercises in more detail. Basically, you use one part of your body to provide resistance against another part. You can do this statically or dynamically. That is, you can simply push your two hands together in front of your chest for the count of thirty, relax, and repeat twenty to forty times, or you can move the two opposing hands in little circles.

Use your imagination here. What are the affordances of the situation you are in? For instance, if you are in a rocking chair, well, by all means rock! If you are in a swivel chair, by all means swivel! If you lying on a bear or sheep skin rug, by all means use the opportunity to do some yoga stretches.

Mute buttons can be dangerous. Before mute buttons, when commercials came on with their blaring sound and flashing senseless images, people would leave the room. Now, some people simply press the mute button and immediately begin texting on their phones or playing a game on their phones. Push the mute button if you must, but *still leave the room.*

CHAPTER 15. WEIGHTING IN LINE.

The Department of Motor Vehicles, getting a ticket, waiting for the theater to open, waiting in cafeteria lines, Disneyland, waiting for rock concert tickets —- these and many more opportunities for exercise present themselves to the busy person. Not only might these opportunities help build your strength and flexibility; given that you are so busy, doing something "useful" while you are waiting will also help make you feel less frustrated.

Of course, if you are in line with others, more possibilities abound. But let's consider the case first where you find yourself in line with strangers. If you have a suitcase, backpack, purse, or attache case, you can certainly use these artifacts in various ways to help build strength in your arms, shoulders, wrists, etc. But you already know that from chapter 10 and the youtube videos.

Now, I realize that in some of these standing in line situations, some of you may find yourself worried about the reactions of strangers when you start exercising. The most elegant approach is steadfastly not to care. But if you cannot manage that, then a shrug and a quick word will do the trick. For example, you catch the eye of someone staring at you and simply say, "Doctor's orders" with a wave of the hand. With a bit of practice, you can utter this line replete with subtext: "What can you do, right?" Or, if you prefer, pretty much the same tones and gestures will work with, "The Wife!" or "The Husband!" No-one wants to really hear about your domestic troubles so that should cut any argument short. Another line you can use is simply, "This is the seventh step. Can't be helped." People will assume you just joined some weird religious cult or are a recovering alcoholic. In either case, they don't want to be responsible for your losing your soul, so they will pretend not to notice.

Of course, some of you might prefer the more confrontational approach. You could say, "I am working hard to stay alive and healthy so as not to be a burden on my family and society. Why aren't you exercising while you're waiting in line?"

If you are about to go to an appointment where you are likely to stand in line and do not *need* to take a backpack or brief case with you, take one *anyway!* You can use these props for curls, wrist curls, triceps exercises, and so on. Obviously, you need to pay attention so as not to run these props into any nearby police officers, TSA personnel, or for that matter, even innocent bystanders (even if it is unlikely that any of them are completely innocent).

If you are in a very long line (for example, let's say you are waiting to get tickets to a Rush concert or one of my book signings), then many of your co-waiters will be happy to exercise with you. You might consider dancing, playing "hot hands" or leading the group in Tai Chi.

Failing that, you can rise on your toes 30-100 times in a row. Or, you can keep your feet still and planted while pressing your thighs toward each other. Then, reverse the tension and try to move your legs outwards. The point is not to move them but to use gravity and friction to provide resistance. You can, of course, keep your place in line while doing jumping jacks, squats, push-ups, knee bends and simply running in place. Here's a general rule: *Any* motion is better than *no* motion. Of course, you will want to consult your friend, Common Sense, to determine what is appropriate to the context. Just do not be too limited by mere embarrassment. If you start exercising, you are making it "okay" for others to do the same. You might be saving their life!

You might think it very unlikely that your exercise would inspire others to do the same. I can tell you from personal experience that this is simply not so. My wife and I used to attend the Ben and Jerry's Folk Festival in Newport Rhode Island with our friends John and Clare-Marie Karat. One of the things I like about outdoor concerts is that you can dance to the music. In general, we had very good luck with the weather at these concerts. One summer day though, the weather did not cooperate at all. Everyone arrived at the concert in rain gear and under umbrellas. It rained pretty steadily, but occasionally, there was a real downpour. There we were: thousands of us, sitting on the damp ground. At first, the combination of umbrellas and rain gear kept us dry. In fact, this combination is pretty good for keeping you dry as you walk to your car from the mall. But I can tell you from personal experience that after an hour, you are pretty much soaked to the skin. Sitting there in soaked clothing, I actually got pretty cold. I decided that I had come to the concert to dance and so that's what I was going to do. I threw down my now useless umbrella, shed my now soaking clothes down to my bathing trunks and began dancing. I discovered that I was actually *warmer* dancing without the wet clothes than I had been before. I became the music and the rain. For the first half hour or so, I was the *only* person dancing. But then, a few more stripped to their bathing clothes and joined me. In another hour, *hundreds* of people were dancing. The music was great, as usual. But dancing to the music provided a much better way for many of us to enjoy the concert than listening while huddling under useless clothes and umbrellas.

CHAPTER 16. LEVERAGING PLACE AND SPACE.

In much of this book, I have tried to convince you not to worry too much about where you are and to take every opportunity to exercise in some fashion or another. This is good advice or I would not have included it. However, now it is time to shift gears. Now, I am going to ask you to try to take advantage of the place and space and see what is *particularly appropriate* to the situation and take advantage of that.

Much as I might like to, I cannot accompany you in every situation. Instead, I am going to give some examples of the idea and you are going to have to see how to apply these in your own life. Since I cannot be there in person, you might find it useful to let your imaginary friends read this chapter and advise you. Failing that, you could also let your real friends work together with you to determine how to find something useful.

Let's suppose that you take a trip to the beach. There are several ways to enjoy being at the beach. You can lay in the sun all day. You can walk along the beach, careful to keep your feet dry (which can be a great option if the beach is littered with jellyfish). Assuming no shark or jellyfish warnings, you can swim in the ocean or body surf or just fight the waves. Ask your imaginary friend which of these is the *only* option that does not increase your fitness.

Or, let's suppose that you go to a museum. You can take the elevator between floors or you can walk up and down the stairs. You can watch your kids interact with all the interactive exhibits or you can join in. You valet park or park the car yourself and walk an extra block or two.

Suppose you go to a ski lodge with some friends. You can decide when to "knock off" for the day and sit in the lounge drinking hot buttered rum. If your friends are still out skiing and you positively cannot ski any more, you might still be able to do an upper body workout that consists of more than moving a pint of ale to your lips.

Suppose you find yourself at a golf course. You have a half hour till tee time. What do you do? Sip a drink to relax or go warm up on the driving range? Are you going to walk the course or take a cart? Unfortunately, some golf courses make you take a cart during certain hours so you might think about this before agreeing to a tee time. Golf courses supposedly do this because of "pace of play" but it is really to make more money. If two people each carry their complete bag of clubs with them, it is just as fast as two people zigging and zagging across the course in a cart unless your course has extremely long green to tee distances. Suppose that you find yourself waiting on every tee shot. How do you spend that time? One common procedure is to stand around and moan and complain about the "slowpokes" in front of you who are slowing everything down. (What you probably cannot see from your vantage point is that they are *also* waiting on every shot). Or, you could use the time to stretch, keep loose, do some squats, rise up on your toes, and enjoy the beautiful surroundings. You make the call. Regardless of where you find yourself, there are always choices that help keep you fit and choices that do not help keep you fit. There are choices that contribute to your mental health and choices that add to your frustration and anger. Your call.

Chapter 17. There is a Season, turn, turn, turn.

Just as particular places and types of spaces lend themselves to certain kinds of activity, so too do different seasons and times of the day. Actually, you probably already knew this. I'm guessing that you seldom walk to work in the summer wearing your snowshoes or in the dead of winter in your bathing suit. Similarly, you don't often try sunbathing at midnight or go digging for earthworms at high noon.

Now is the time to extend that intelligent behavior into thinking about how to make use of time as your friend when it comes to staying alive and strong through exercise!

At the broadest scale, age plays a part in exercise. I have one friend in his sixties who plays rugby. But that is rather unusual. Most people tend to start avoiding full contact sports after 40. It isn't that you cannot do it. It just takes a bit longer for the broken bones to heal. Hiking, jogging, biking, tennis, golf, racquetball, swimming, dancing and rowing are just a few of the many sports and activities that most people can enjoy their whole life. For more tips on choosing a sport and making the most of it, you will undoubtedly want to read my book, The Winning Weekend Warrior.

At the next level, there are the seasons. And, by the way, at least in the US northeast and upper midwest, there are not *four* seasons, but *six*. The idea that there are four equally long seasons is absurd. In Westchester County New York, for example, true spring is usually only about three weeks from the end of April to the third week in May. Summer however, lasts from May through September. All those spectacular autumn colors peak for another three weeks. By the end of October, that is gone. So, what comes next? Winter? No way! Next comes "The Dead Time" which takes all of November and most of December. There is typically no color and no snow either. It is cold, windy and wet. Finally, winter arrives and it can take up the last week of December as well as all of January, February and most of March. Finally, it stops snowing but no new growth appears. This is "The Waiting" and is another season with lots of nasty weather.

Various exercises and activities and sports are best suited to the different seasons. For example, a nice day in Spring or Autumn is a great time to go for a long walk or hike. Winter also provides opportunities for that but clearly you need to dress appropriately and check the weather forecast. You can actually burn more calories on a winter walk because of the cold and extra weight. If you get a chance to trudge through the snow, so much the better. Similarly, hot summer weather lends itself to running along the surf. Letting the waves chase you, running through water, body surfing and keeping your balance while waves smack against you are all great fun. Most localities and local clubs organize activities for various times of year. Whether it is going to a haunted house, participating in an Easter Egg hunt, or going to Mardi Gras or Beltane celebrations, you can find fun ways to challenge yourself in every season.

In a similar way, the day of the week and the time of day also inspire you to be active in different ways. Maybe it is part of your "normal" routine, Monday through Friday to circle the parking lot three times to get a spot close to the front door of your destination. What if, instead, you just parked farther away and walked? Maybe you would make it to your office building, precinct or grocery store entrance just as quickly.

Maybe you are at work and your company, like most companies, has decided that it is more "cost-effective" and "efficient" to get rid of all office support and just let everyone do their own typing, printing, copying, scheduling, etc. In that absurd but common case, you will be spending time waiting during a copying job. You might have to wait to use the espresso machine. In these cases, you can do some exercises while you wait. And, no, they are unlikely to fire you. Or, let's put it this way. If you are a star performer and they fire you because you are exercising (and saving them medical costs), then, they are a sinking ship.

Maybe at home, you often make yourself a microwave dinner. Okay, but what do you do during the 3-5 minutes it takes for dinner to cook? You do not *have* to sit down and watching soul-wrenching, frightening news about things you cannot influence. Instead, you could exercise. Lift your legs; swivel your hips; pace; dance a dance you make up on the spot. Tune in to your body and you will see it *wants* to move. And, if you tune in, it will hopefully also tell you how *not* to move. If you just got a double knee replacement, you probably want to ask your doctor before doing the twist, for example. If you are 80 and wearing high heels, yes, take it easy. Be reasonable but be *active* at whatever level makes sense for you.

And, after dinner, you might decide it is time to wash the week's worth of dishes you have been letting accumulate. Fine and dandy but — remember that this is also an opportunity to be more active. For example, when you are done washing the dishes and are now drying them, you could stand in front of the cupboard and dry a dish and then place the dish in the cupboard. Or, you could, while you are drying the dish, also walk around that granite island. It takes no more time but it is better for you.If you have a baby strapped to your back or chest, so much the better. The baby was about to wake up and scream because you *weren't* walking anyway. You may as well outthink them and start walking before they scream. After all, you are the parent here. You can, with a little thought, probably arrange to play music while you wash and dry dishes (or do other housework) and this will help inspire you to move as well.

We now have a central vacuum system, but when we had a hand-held model, I used it to build up strength for my golf swing. Rather than push and pull the vacuum cleaner toward me and away again (which is what most people do), instead, I moved the vacuum cleaner in a line parallel with my shoulders. If you are a right-handed golfer, you especially need to make your left arm strong, so I would often vacuum by holding the handle in my left hand only and pushing and pulling it in the manner described.

CHAPTER 18. PEOPLE NEED PEOPLE.

Studies indicate what should be rather obvious. People tend to be and become like those they are with. This does not mean you should drop all your current friends immediately and chum around only with elite athletes. No. Do it gradually over the course of days or weeks. Hopefully, it is clear I am kidding. But there is some truth to this outrageous suggestion. At least *some* of your friends should hopefully be active people. If everyone you hang around with is a couch potato, that is going to make it that much harder for you to stay in shape. If the people you are with do not support your exercise efforts, that will tend to undermine those efforts over time.

On the other hand, other people can be a great source of encouragement instead. Find and cherish people who will work with you to help your exercise efforts. The same goes for diet as well. If you hang out with folks who tend to have drinks before dinner, a couple bottles of wine with steak for dinner, and Irish coffee and pecan pie for dessert, then, it will be difficult to keep looking like your true and athletic self. Generally, when people go out to dinner, either no-one has dessert or everyone does. The same is pretty much true with healthy foods as well. A whole book could be written on the social effects of eating. But that is a different book.

For now, let's try to stay focused on the topic at hand which is gaining encouragement from others. Hanging out with people who like physical activity will go a long ways toward helping you stay more active. But do not feel as though you are only a passive participant. Even if you are with a group of people who eschew physical activity in general, you can still take a leadership role and convince, cajole, encourage, sell, and persuade others to be active at this particular time. People on television commercials convince total strangers to buy all kinds of useless expensive crap. It should be much easier for you to convince them to do something that is both fun and healthy than that should spend half their paycheck on a whizzy gizmo or a drug that causes people's livers to explode.

Of course, people you don't even know can be inspirational as well. Some people find it helpful to put a picture of their favorite athlete on the refrigerator door. Others find that watching their favorite sports figure or team can be inspiring. Still other people find reading about sports heroes motivational. Movies about underdogs or people who overcome handicaps to be successful can offer another source of motivation.

When groups of people get together to do something, there is often a division of labor. This provides you an opportunity. Volunteer! If a group of people is playing cards in the teak paneled den and someone needs to go into the kitchen to bring in the next round of drinks, volunteer! Sure, it doesn't expend a lot of calories but it is better for your body than staying at the table. If someone needs to go kill a wooly mammoth to provide for the upcoming feast, be the one to volunteer. You'd be surprised how many calories can be expended in tracking and slaying a single mammoth. Do that every day for a year and you'll be surprised how much fitter you will feel at the end of the year. Now, I understand that you may live in a climate where wooly mammoths are actually quite rare. But you can do the translation into something that is appropriate for your situation. Even if you volunteer to drive to the 7-11 to get ice, you will have to walk to the car, walk to the store from the parking lot, search for the ice (watch out for mammoths —- this is where they hang out!), carry the ice to the counter, fish out your credit card, carry the ice to the car, and so on.

You may have watched Serena Williams or Azarenka play tennis. When events are going south, these top athletes appeal to their imaginary friends. They stand facing away from the court and get some sage advice and counsel from these imaginary friends. They do not have a patent on this. You too can have imaginary friends. In fact, you may well have had imaginary friends when you were a kid. Somehow, over the years, you and your imaginary friends have probably lost touch. I am not trying to assign blame here. It may well have mostly been the fault of the imaginary friend. It might have mostly been you yourself who failed to keep up the contact. But whoever was more to fault is not the issue. Let bygones be bygones and do whatever it takes to win back your imaginary friend or friends.

If you prefer electronic friends, of course, you can turn to them. I find it kind of fun to wear a fit bit (@)or similar device to keep track of steps and calories. This can help *remind* you, for example, that it is not a *law* (at least in most states) that you must sit during an entire television show. You *are* allowed to stand. In fact, you can even walk around. The actors on television will not be offended. In fact, they will probably be happy because you will be healthier and their tax burden will be lower. Having a fit bit (@) or similar device can encourage you by showing how many steps you can actually take while watching CSI Miami Vice or Psych. In fact, you do not have to stick to walking during a television show. If you are lucky enough to be watching Psych, you can emulate Spencer and his energetic fake "trances" in order to get a more full body workout.

While dwelling on electronics overjoys me, let's return to imaginary friends. What kind of imaginary friend would be most motivating to you? Would they be an encourager? A curmudgeon or a little of both? Or, would an angry in-law work better? Or, perhaps a magical animal? A dragon? A wolf? A wise Yoda like character? And, how could they best encourage you?

Of course, when it comes to real people, one of the fine ways for people to help each other is through competitions. Who can walk the most steps each day or each week? Who can climb the most stairs? Who can convince the most friends to buy their own copy of this ebook? Who can lift the most total weight during the course of a week? Who can juggle the greatest number of balls or rotating flaming chain saws? Actually, maybe you should save that competition for your imaginary friends to work out among themselves. Either that or use imaginary chain saws.

When it comes to real people, it is good to remember that not everyone is blessed with perfect health. There may well be people in your area who need your physical help with daily tasks. If you are super busy, it might be difficult to volunteer for many hours, but perhaps you could spare the time to mow someone's lawn, carry their groceries upstairs, or shovel the snow off their driveway. Doing something that helps others may give you an opportunity to help you stay fit but studies show that doing something good for others is also good for you psychologically as well.

CHAPTER 19. LAYER UPON LAYER.

The word "LAYER" is mean to be an acronym to help you recall the facets of fitness and to remind you to look for opportunities. What does "LAYER" stand for? It stands for five role models.

L is for "Lineman" in American football to remind you of Strength. Strength is not just about showing off. Strength can help you in emergencies. It can help keep you from falling if you trip. It means you can open a jar of pickles without swearing a blue streak. It is helpful in just about every sport you can imagine. Well, at least it is helpful in every sport I can imagine including shuffleboard and croquet. Look for opportunities to improve your strength. You can do this by pushing, lifting, pulling against resistance. That resistance can be provided by weights or machines as in a gym, but it can also be provided by strong stable objects or by your own body or by your workout partner. It *cannot* safely be provided by pushing against a large plate glass window. So, even when it comes to strength, you need to use some common sense. Apparently, common sense is not quite so common as one might imagine. In our gym, there is a sign that says, "Do not bounce weights against the mirror." So, in case you do go to a gym and they have forgotten to post that useful sign, you should avoid bouncing weights against the mirrors anyway.

A is for "Acrobat." An acrobat is meant to remind you of balance. You can (and should) find safe ways to practice balance every day. If you do that from now until you are 110 years old, you are much less likely to fall in your 11th, 12th, 13th decades and beyond. But, here again, use some common sense. Do not start practicing your balance by walking a tightrope suspended over the Grand Canyon. You might try standing on one foot when you are brushing your teeth or waiting for the microwave to beep. But balance is also meant to remind you of having balance in your life as well. Do not make it all about increasing the take home pay of your CEO from $15,500,505 to $15,500,525 by missing your kid's school play or neglecting your own body's welfare. Needless to say, the CEO will try to convince you that his or her salary is the most important thing in life. They won't put it in precisely those terms, of course. They will talk about the competition, the customers, the advancement of humanity, the bottom line, and so on, but actually, they are talking about their power to get you to do what they want. After all, if *everyone* in the company stayed fit, the company would be better off as would their customers, but they would not feel quite so powerful as when they are convincing you, quite literally, to give up your life for theirs.

Y is for "Yogi" — those incredibly flexible people who keep celebrating "Nama's Day" all year round. Yoga itself is a great workout, but even if you cannot always take an hour class, take a few and/or get some videos so as to get some clue as to the right way to do certain moves. Personally, I like the Rodney Yee videos. But even if you never get into yoga or learn how to breathe through your eyelids or relax your liver, you need to keep working on flexibility throughout your life. Do not *overdo* the stretching though. The point is not to "win" but to stay flexible. If you do go to an actual yoga class, if you are a beginner, please do not try to stretch as far as people who are younger or who have been taking yoga forever. Just stretch to the point where you feel it, not to the point of snapping. And, in reality, what they are saying is not "Nama's Day" but "Namaste" which means, roughly speaking, "I acknowledge the divinity in you." To my way of thinking, this is a really nice sentiment and well worth repeating. Why? Because everyone living *is* extremely complex and beautiful in their own way.

E is for Enjoyment of Life. Try to practice thinking of sports and exercise of all kinds as ways to enhance your enjoyment of life and feel more fully alive. We are *animals*, not plants. I have nothing against plants. I love my garden, but *our* ancestors took a different path. That path is the path of movement. You know in your heart that you feel a lot more alive when you are walking or dancing or playing tennis than when you are sitting on a couch. Whether it comes to exercise or eating right, it is not about "sin"; it is about physics and physiology. If you move as we evolved to do for a billion years, you will burn more calories, be more fit, and almost certainly enjoy life more. Unfortunately, so many people have been conditioned to think of exercise as a chore or a duty or something one really must do when one gets around to it, that the *enjoyment* that should be a natural part of any kind of movement is overlooked.

Please watch your language! Avoid saying, "Oh, I'd better do some sit-ups" or "Now, I have to run." No! It is an honor and a privilege to be able to do these things. You probably no longer recall how much joy you experienced when you first learned to crawl and then walk and then jump. These are *wonderful* and *joyful* activities! They are not chores. Remember that.

R is for "Runner" to remind you that you want to keep your cardiovascular fitness as well. It doesn't mean you have to run, although if you are capable of running, it is one way to keep cardiovascular fitness. Others include cross country skiing, biking, walking, tennis, racquetball, squash, square dancing, ballroom dancing, hiking, snow shoveling, climbing, rowing, wrestling and martial arts training. Of course, there are machines in many gyms that enable you to do one or more of these activities. But there are opportunities to walk, at least, almost every day. Some degree of consistency is very important here. If people sit on the couch and watch TV for hours at a time every day and then go out and shovel snow for an hour, they may indeed die of a heart attack. We could debate whether it was actually shoveling snow or TV that killed them, but we cannot argue that with the person who died. That's what it means to die. If you die, you won't be able to win any more arguments. In fact, rumor has it that even losing an argument can be more fun than dying. It is something to avoid. So, as I've already mentioned, make sure you check with your medical practitioners about your exercise and increase cardio work gradually. Don't try to "make up for lost time" by running a marathon your first month after getting inspired by my book.

CHAPTER 20. OH, YES, YOU CAN!

Oh, but it is so easy to fall into old habits; to procrastinate; to generate excuses; to laugh about the whole thing; to claim you want to enjoy life today rather than be endlessly worried about tomorrow; to say it is just "normal" to degenerate with age. You and I, dear reader, could play that game forever. I could come up with additional ways you could exercise and keep fit and live longer and you could come up with more excuses about why you cannot do this, that or the other thing, all the while insisting that of course, you know that *in principle,* it's a good idea to exercise and that you probably *will* exercise once your kids, Suzie and Lynda are a little older or your job is a little easier or your household is a little more organized, or your taxes are done or, or, or, or....Well, this isn't a game. At least, this isn't a game I am playing with you. It's your life we are talking about here. And, if you are sick, incapacitated or dead, I guarantee you that your kids will not like it, your job will suffer, your household will be less organized and your taxes will be later than ever.

The key is to start and to start now. Another key is to start small. You do not have to leap from sedentary to Olympic athlete in one day. In fact, that isn't even recommended, at least not in this book. Small steps. Start with something doable and then actually do it. Perhaps you really do want to start jogging. Great. If you don't have time to go for a four mile run today, put on your jogging suit. Tomorrow, put on your jogging suit and jog from one end of your driveway to the other. You get the picture.

Understand that being in shape and eating right is not about being "moral" or "sinful." It is purely about physics, chemistry, biology and psychology. It is *science.* If you consistently eat more calories than you expend then you will gain weight. If you consistently burn more calories than you eat, you will lose weight. How much can that effect be moderated by excuses or promises or cajoling or humor? Zero. Yes, zero.

If you stretch and move your limbs through their complete range of motion every day, you will stay relatively flexible all through your life. If you sit in the car on the way to work; sit at your computer all day; sit in the car on the way home; and then sit and watch TV all evening, you will lose your flexibility. Do you know how much that loss of mobility will be affected by whether you have *really good* excuses versus having *really lame* excuses? Zero. Yes. Zero. Compare two situations. Situation one: You eat more calories than you burn up and do not come up with any excuse whatsoever. Situation two: You eat more calories than you burn up and come up with what everyone agrees is the very best excuse in the world! Yay! Do you know what? The amount of weight gain will *precisely the same.* I am *not* saying you should feel guilty. I am saying do not *bother* to feel guilty. Do not bother to feel virtuous either. It's irrelevant. Staying fit is a function of what you actually *do.* It is completely unimportant what excuses you come up with.

There is no magic abacus, iPad, or Android keeping track of your excuses. That is not all bad news either. Since it is merely science, you can save all that mental energy that you put into justifying what you are doing to the magic abacus and instead put your imagination to work finding ways to motivate yourself to slowly, but inexorably to do a little more in the way of being healthier. How that plays out precisely will depend on you. After all, you know you better than I do.

It is conceivable, for instance, that you care about your kids. I have already mentioned that they are likely to be a lot happier if you die at a ripe old age rather than keel over in your prime. In addition, you are setting a role model for them *all the time.* If you are working virtually all the time and caring nothing about your health, then regardless of what you say to them about the rules of health or how many soccer games you drive them to, a loud clear message comes through and that message is that your life is not a joy but a job or a series of jobs. They may be fit while they are in organized athletics in school, but later in life, they will have your model in their heads to fall back on. And that will speak much more clearly and loudly than any words you or their health teacher speak to them. *Your* being a middle aged couch potato will surely increase the chances that they will end up the same way.

Of course, there are no guarantees. It is also possible, though far less likely, that they will see you being "responsible" day after day and living for them apparently without regard to your own physical needs and spending so much time in the "Rat Race" that they will rebel so far against spending their own life in that endless Rat Race that they will decide to drop out of that whole scene way earlier than you would have imagined possible.

The bottom line is that if you won't do it for yourself, at least do it for your kids. Show them that it is okay and in fact, crucial, to take some time for your own physical and emotional needs and stay fit. After all, I'm not saying everyone needs to be spending hours a day at maximum heart rate. I am just saying it will benefit you and your friends and family to give some *thought* to changing your routines, little by little, to include more cardio, stretching and weight bearing exercise.

Speaking of giving thought to things, when you are changing habits, it helps to think ahead. So, for example, if you have a reserved parking space near the entrance and you decide to park a block away so as to give yourself some minimal exercise, before you take off for work, you would do well to visualize yourself driving into the parking lot and thinking, "Hey, wait. I want to park a block away!" Then, when you actually arrive at work, you are much more likely to remember to give yourself that block walk there and block walk back. If you do forget the first day and pull into your space because you are spaced out, just check the rearview mirror, back out and return to where you meant to park. Yes, you might arrive at work three minutes later. And don't worry. If civilization falls because you got to work three minutes later, maybe it wasn't worth saving.

Of course, the use of physical reminders can also be powerful and probably more effective than visualized mental reminders. When I managed a research project on the psychology of aging at Harvard Medical School in the 1970's, one of my bosses was Dr. Nancy Waugh, a fairly famous experimental psychologist and a memory expert. I had told her about an interesting book I thought she would enjoy but I kept forgetting to bring the book in to work. Every day I remembered — but only after I got to work. Finally, I challenged her. "Nancy," I said, "You are one of the world experts in memory. You should have a technique for helping me remember." Without pausing, Nancy opened up her purse silently, brought out a small piece of string and tied it around my finger. I said, "That's it? Tie a piece of string around my finger?" Well, the next day, I did bring the book into work. She was a brilliant experimentalist, but she also had a practical bent. So, if you want to remind yourself of some plan to exercise, I heartily recommend putting some physical cues in your environment to remind yourself. If you want to do something as simple as make your grip stronger, get a rubber ball or a grip from a sporting goods store and then put it in plain sight on your desk or on top of the TV remote control. Don't hide it in a drawer.

If you want to recall that you can use your backpack as a weight training aid, put a little sticker or symbol on it. If you want to remind yourself that the Amendment to the US Constitution that required people to sit still during television programs has been repealed, then put a sticker on your TV remote or on the edge of the TV itself. And then use that as a cue to actually walk around the room. Small steps. At first, just walk around during commercials. Later, during advanced television viewing, you will find that you can pace during shows without losing the flow. Get creative. If you are watching *Lost,* you can walk when they walk. If you are watching *Game of Thrones,* you can pretend to slay when they slay. If you are watching *Dancing with the Stars,* you will *not* want to try everything they are doing full tilt. But you could join in at the level that is safe and appropriate. As I say, that Amendment requiring US citizens to stay on their butts while watching TV has been repealed. Use that hard won freedom. Get your spouse into it. Get your kids into it. Get your whole extended family into it. People dance at weddings. Why not at Thanksgiving and for every Holiday? Why not invent a dance craze for "President's Day" and why not dance with a sweetheart on Valentine's Day?

When I was in graduate school at Michigan, one of our professors was originally from Japan. While still a graduate student in Japan, he had been terribly excited to read about Skinner's work on positive reinforcement. In an article which he had painstakingly translated from English, Skinner had described how a rat would press a lever and receive a food pellet in response. Excited to replicate this, this Japanese grad student invited the whole psychology department to watch how a rat could be so trained. They did not have the automatic dispensers but he was ready with a knife to cut some rice cake for the rat when it pressed the lever. The whole department watched while the grad student was ready for that first level press. Everyone watched. And watched. And waited. And waited. And gradually drifted out. Since this was Japan where people are polite, it took a good long time, but eventually they all left. Only the faithful graduate student himself stayed, waiting for the rat to press the lever. And finally, after two days, it did.

The next month, the second issue of the journal came and the then graduate student learned about "successive approximations." Pressing levers is not something rats normally do. If you want to get them to press levers, you do not wait until they press a lever and then reinforce them. Well, not unless you have the patience of Job. You begin by reinforcing them when they are in the same *half* of the cage as the lever. Then you only reinforce them when they are *near* the lever. Then, you only reinforce them when they *touch* the lever. Then, you only reinforce them when they stand on their hind legs and touch the lever. *Finally,* you begin reinforcing them only for pressing the lever (which at this point can be easily automated). Small steps.

This is a vital concept for teaching children. At first, you praise them just for touching a washcloth; then you reinforce them for touching it to their face; then you reinforce them for pushing it on their face with some force. Eventually, you will only reinforce them if they do a good job of cleaning their face. But you do not *begin* by only praising them when they do a good job of cleaning their face! Most parents are hip to this but some actually expect immediate perfection. Small steps.

Less often do adults apply this same technique to themselves. Reward yourself when you change *a little bit* in the direction of incorporating some exercise into your daily routine. Do not wait for you to change from a couch potato into a rock hard body before rewarding yourself. Remember. It is about science, not about how "good" or "bad" you are as a person. The *science* shows that you will do better if you reward yourself for progress toward your goal. Don't wait till you lose 50 pounds or run a marathon before you get any tangible or social reward. Small steps.

One last thing about motivation. In this book, I have given some suggestions about what has worked *for me*. You have your own set of constraints, preferences, and contexts. You might be older, younger, living in a hotter or colder climate, etc. I guarantee that you can do *something* and then something else differently. You need to use your own creativity to figure out what those somethings are as well as what kind of rewards work best for changing your behavior over time. Apart from physical benefits, the approach I am suggesting here is above all, an exercise in creative problem solving. I am asking you to overcome your habitual ways of thinking about physical and social situations; to look at the artifacts and tools in your environment and open up your mind as to what they can be used for. In particular, look at these things in terms of how they can be safely and productively used to enhance your strength, flexibility, balance, and endurance. If you do this consistently, you will not only reap substantial physical benefits; you will also find yourself in a much more inventive frame of mind when it comes to everything in life. Tools have an intended use. But they can also be *appropriated* for *novel* uses. Practice appropriate appropriation, as it were, and you will begin to see life in much more interesting and inventive terms.

I would love to hear about any of your own inventions and innovations along these lines. If you got something good out of this book and found it helpful, naturally, I would appreciate it if you feel like writing a review to help others also become healthier and happier. In any case, "live long and prosper."

ABOUT THE AUTHOR

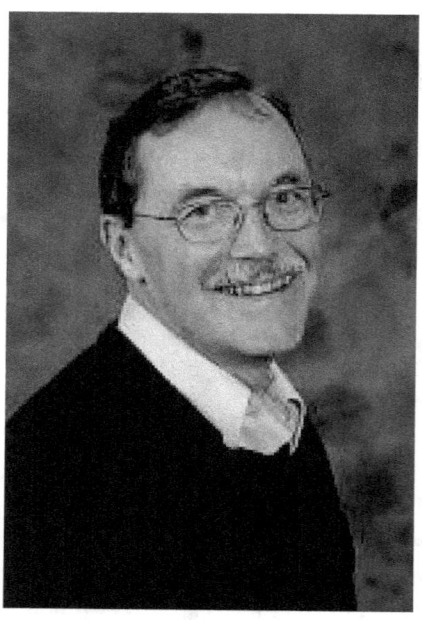

JOHN CHARLES THOMAS has over 200 publications and talks on various topics in the psychology of aging, artificial intelligence and human-computer interaction. He lives in Solana Beach, California and is principle of !Problem Solving International, a consulting company focusing on finding, formulating, and solving complex problems. You can often find him on the golf course, the tennis courts, the gym or walking along the beach. Learn more about John at https://www.amazon.com/author/truthtableBlogs include:

http://johncharlesthomas.sportsblog.com

https://petersironwood.wordpress.com

BOOKS BY JOHN CHARLES THOMAS:

THE WINNING WEEKEND WARRIOR: HOW TO SUCCEED AT GOLF, TENNIS, BASEBALL, FOOTBALL, BASKETBALL, HOCKEY, VOLLEYBALL, BUSINESS,LIFE, ETC.

TURING'S NIGHTMARES: SCENARIOS AND SPECULATIONS ON "THE SINGULARITY"

ONE LAST THING...

If you enjoyed this book or found it useful I'd be very grateful if you would post a short review on Amazon. Your support really does make a difference and I read all the reviews personally so I use your feedback to make this book even better.

I realize that describing movements with words is difficult. Be sure to search for my demonstration videos on youtube.com. Using my name and "Fit in Bits" as search terms should get you there quickly. By the way, you will find many other useful videos on moves for exercise and sports on youtube.com.

Thanks again for your support! Live long and prosper!